Walkin' the Dog, Denver

By M. A. Savage

FALCON®

Guilford, Connecticut

An Imprint of The Globe Pequot Press

Copyright © 2001 by The Globe Pequot Press

All rights reserved. No part of this book may be reproduced or transmitted in any form by any means, electronic or mechanical, including photocopying and recording, or by any information storage and retrieval system, except as may be expressly permitted by the 1976 Copyright Act or by the publisher. Requests for permission should be made in writing to The Globe Pequot Press, P.O. Box 480, Guilford, CT 06437.

Falcon and FalconGuide are registered trademarks of The Globe Pequot Press.

Cover photo by Bob Winsett
Cover design by Libby Kingsbury
Text design, page layout, and map design by Lisa Reneson
Interior photos by M. A. Savage
Photo on p. 1 was taken at Delaney Farm, p. 117 at Frazer Meadow, and p. 153 at Cherry Creek State Park.

Library of Congress Cataloging-in-Publication Data

Savage, M. A.
    Walkin' the dog: Denver/by M.A. Savage.—1st ed.
        p. cm.
    ISBN 1-56044-933-0
    1. Dog walking—Colorado—Denver Region—Guidebooks. 2. Denver Region (Colo.)—Guidebooks. I. Title: Walking the dog. II. Title.

SF427.46.S28 2001
636.7—dc21   2001023792

Manufactured in the United States of America
First Edition/First Printing

Dedication

This book is dedicated to Gold Rush
and all the other dogs who,
as loyal and uncomplaining companions,
have enhanced our enjoyment
of Colorado's spectacular landscape.

Contents

Introduction   viii

The Metro Denver Greenbelt Loop   1

High Line Canal
Walk 1 Platte Canyon Reservoir   11
Walk 2 Highlands Ranch   15
Walk 3 Writer Vista Park   18
Walk 4 DeKoevend Open Space Park   22
Walk 5 Orchard Road to Long Road   26
Walk 6 Orchard Road to Belleview Avenue   30
Walk 7 Dahlia Street to Belleview Avenue   35
Walk 8 Dahlia Street to East Quincy Avenue   38
Walk 9 Colorado Boulevard to East Quincy Avenue   40
Walk 10 Colorado Boulevard to East Hampden Avenue   43
Walk 11 Eisenhower Park to I–25   46
Walk 12 Bible Park   49
Walk 13 Potomac Street, Aurora Greenhouse,
           and Flower Garden   52
Walk 14 DeLaney Farm   56

South Platte River Greenway
Walk 15 Discovery Pavilion   60
Walk 16 Discovery Pavilion, River Route   64
Walk 17 Chatfield State Park   68
Walk 18 South Platte Park   71
Walk 19 Ruby Hill Park Area   76
Walk 20 Confluence Park to City of Cuernavaca Park   80
Walk 21 East Eighty-Eighth Avenue to McKay Road   85
Walk 22 Adams County Regional Park   89

Cherry Creek Greenway

Walk 23 Confluence Park   93

Walk 24 Alamo Placita Park to Speer Gazebo   97

Walk 25 Four Mile House Park   101

Walk 26 Cherry Creek and High Line Canal Intersection   105

Sand Creek Regional Greenway

Walk 27 Star K Ranch Open Space   109

Walk 28 Sand Creek at Bluff Lake   112

The Foothills 117

Walk 29 Rock Creek Farm   120

Walk 30 Bear Creek Lake Park   123

Walk 31 Standley Lake Regional Park (South)   126

Walk 32 Standley Lake Regional Park (North)   129

Walk 33 Van Bibber Park   132

Walk 34 Crown Hill Lake Open Space Park   135

Walk 35 Matthew-Winters Park   138

Walk 36 Apex Trail 141

Walk 37 Lair o' the Bear Park 145

Walk 38 Frazer Meadow 149

Dog Heavens 153

Walk 39 Chatfield State Park 156

Walk 40 Cherry Creek State Park 159

Walk 41 Elk Meadow Park 162

Walk 42 Highlands Ranch 165

Walk 43 Washington Park 167

Appendix A: Park Agencies and Organizations 172

Appendix B: Dog-Friendly Organizations 174

Appendix C: Annual Dog Events 177

Acknowledgements 179

About the Author 180

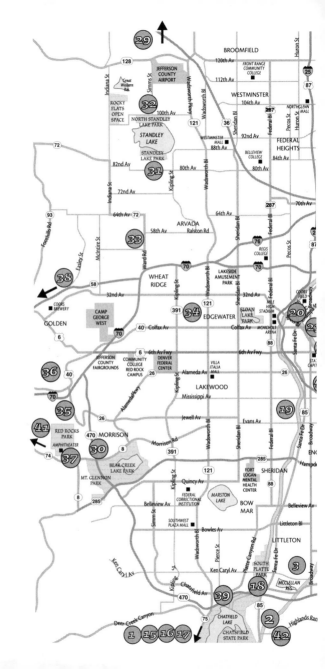

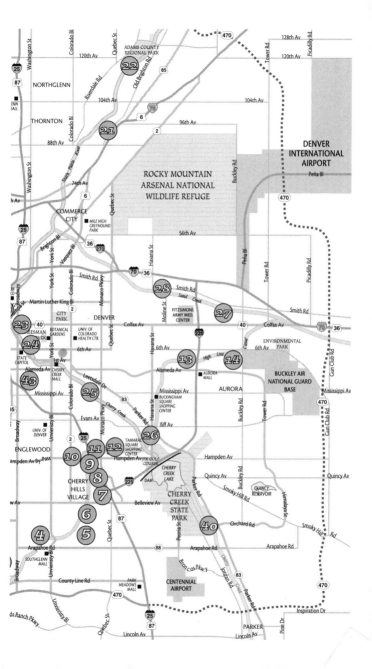

Introduction

very morning for some ten years, Gold Rush, a gentle and lovable golden retriever, would wake me up. He came to my bed, nudged my face with his nose, licked me if the nudge hadn't roused me, and thus told me that the sun was up, the magpies were quarreling in the cottonwoods, and it was time for our morning walk.

We lived near the High Line Canal, and this is where we walked. This canal, built in the Denver area in the 1880s for irrigation, became in the 1970s the metro area's first recreational greenbelt. Today Gold Rush is gone but the High Line Canal constitutes one leg of an expanding system of greenways that will in the early years of the twenty-first century create a 100-plus-mile greenbelt loop around central Denver, a recreational feature not available in any other large U.S. city.

Walkin' the Dog, Denver is the first guide that pinpoints the best portions of these greenbelts for you and your dog to walk, as well as other prime areas in the foothills and along little-known green corridors in the city and the suburbs. These interconnected, multiuse trails offer an incredible opportunity to walk amid nature and wildlife—with your best friend—yet not travel very far afield.

In this guide you will find the most dog-friendly trails—those that provide shade and an opportunity for your companion to take a swim. Walks off the greenbelts follow creekside trails or circumnavigate lakes, explore open-space areas, and visit municipal, county, and state parks where dogs are welcome. The final section of the book is devoted to "dog heavens," public lands where your dog can frolic off leash.

In addition, each walk lists trip access information, as well as amenities and interesting features in the area of each outing. Detailed maps accompany each walk, illustrating the recommended route. You'll also find a map legend at the end of this introduction.

The walks were selected with both you and your canine companion in mind. They offer an escape from congestion and urban noise while providing panoramic views and access to historical sites for you to enjoy. For the comfort and enjoyment of your canine companion, hikes on rough, rocky terrain were avoided in favor of those on packed dirt or aggregate. Shade and access to water were sought-after amenities for your dog.

I continue to walk often on the High Line with Gold Rush's successor, but I still think of my first canine hiking companion. I remember how he sniffed out interesting scents and how he wallowed luxuriantly in the cool water, then—dripping and happy—shook the water from his hide and gave me an impromptu shower whether I wanted one or not. These are the kinds of memories I hope *Walkin' the Dog, Denver* will help you create for yourself.

Walkin' with Man's (and Woman's) Finest Companion

Dogs have been companions to humans for some 10,000 years, since they were first domesticated for use in hunting. Today they're still reliable hunting partners, although most of us choose them as our hiking, jogging, and walking friends. They don't complain if we walk too fast or too slow; they don't chide that we have gone too far or taken a wrong turn. In a pinch, a dog can assist in helping or getting help if something goes wrong during the walk.

But taking your dog along on a walk involves more than making room for him in the car, not forgetting the leash, and remembering to stock up on extra water and a dish from which your friend can drink. Some pretrip preparation, such as making sure your dog is fit for an excursion, will make for a more pleasant outing. Dogs, like humans, can become athletes through training and conditioning. A "couch potato" dog, like a "couch potato" human needs to start out slowly on easy trails to build up stamina and endurance. If you hike with your pet, a working knowledge of canine first aid is recommended.

You need to teach your dog not to chase wildlife. It will add to your enjoyment of the walk and if you can prevent your pet, with a voice command, from disappearing into the brush (and getting lost) while pursuing a deer or squirrel. Since most of the walks in this guide are in urban areas, local regulations require that your dog be on a leash, usually no longer than 6 feet.

In general, a well-behaved dog is welcome on the path. This guide does not include any walks in wilderness areas or other spots where the presence of canines is severely restricted. Excursions to Rocky Mountain National Park are thus not included, since pets are not allowed on the trails or in the backcountry there. Pets are allowed in most campgrounds, however, including those in Rocky Mountain National Park. Your dog is also welcome on U.S. Bureau of Land Management (BLM) land and in federal forests. However, hikes in Colorado BLM lands are not included in this guide, because there are none in the immediate Denver metro area.

If you do venture out with your dog to BLM-administered lands, you might like to know that the bureau has no specific policies regarding dogs, except that they be under control by the owner and not pose a nuisance to others. This rule also applies to pets hiking with owners in national forests. State parks have varying policies on admitting dogs; it would be wise to check beforehand. For example, Roxborough State Park in the southwest Denver metro area does not allow pets at any time, nor does the portion of the Colorado Trail that goes through Waterton Canyon.

In the appendices of this book you'll find a list of addresses and telephone numbers for municipal, county, special district, state, and federal agencies. Also listed are special events and organizations for canines and human companions.

Whether you're a newcomer to Denver or a native, this guide will enhance your enjoyment and knowledge of the city and its immediate environs as you walk with your pet.

Pet Protocol

🐾 Never leave your dog locked in your car during warm weather. Temperatures in a vehicle with the windows rolled down only several inches can quickly reach 150 degrees, causing your pet to suffer heat stroke or convulsions.

🐾 If you're walking the High Line Canal or exploring the foothills with your dog, make sure to check paws for burrs and his coat for ticks, which can cause Rocky Mountain tick fever.

🐾 Do not let your dog drink directly from lakes or streams; this water is often subject to bacterial contamination. Bring along fresh water for your pet instead—and don't forget a bowl that he can drink from!

🐾 In urban areas and parks, clean up after your pet. Carry a few plastic bags with you. Denver parks and Jefferson County Open Space areas usually have bag dispensers and trash receptacles for disposal of the waste.

🐾 Do not let pets swim near beaches or in reservoirs.

🐾 Keep pets away from other animals. Parks, open-space areas, and public lands are home to a variety of wildlife. Respect their natural habitat and keep pets away from nests and burrows. It is against Colorado state law for dogs to harass wildlife.

🐾 Seek out dog training areas where your pet can be trained and exercised without a leash (see Dog Heavens).

🐾 Consider sending your new companion to obedience class.

🐾 Remember that you are the leader your dog looks to for direction. Be a good leader by building trust, friendship, and respect.

🐾 If you make training and exercising fun for your pet, your dog will listen and learn.

Map Legend

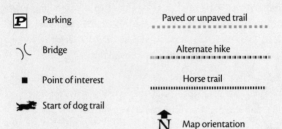

P   Parking

)(Bridge

■   Point of interest

   Start of dog trail

❖ ❖ ❖   The dog trail

Paved or unpaved trail

Alternate hike

Horse trail

N   Map orientation

The Metro Denver Greenbelt Loop

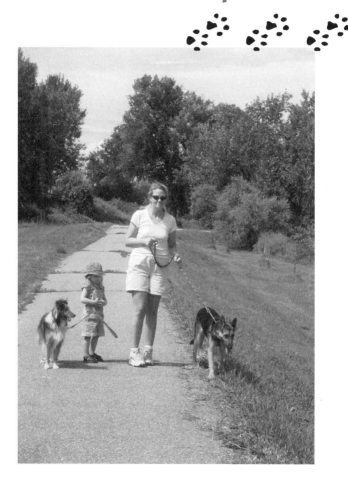

The Metro Denver Greenbelt Loop

When conversations turn to the outdoor lifestyle, the city of Denver usually crops up. Not only is Denver the gateway to the Colorado Rocky Mountains, but its metrowide, multiuse greenbelt system is unique in the country as well. This continually expanding system offers a 100-plus-mile loop of interconnected trails around the metropolitan area, providing a regional amenity unknown to any other major U.S. city. This system includes four greenbelts: the High Line Canal, the South Platte River Greenway, the Cherry Creek Greenway, and the Sand Creek Regional Greenway.

High Line Canal

The High Line Canal is the oldest trail and greenbelt in the loop. It was built in the 1880s by a land development company to attract settlers to the parched prairie by providing water to the land. Considered a marvel of Victorian engineering, the canal diverted water from the South Platte River as the river emerged from the mountains southwest of Denver, then carried the water soley by gravity. This feat was accomplished by building the channel to follow the descending contour of the prairie as it slopes away from the foothills. The resulting channel follows the high line of the topography in giant, meandering loops. In its time as an irrigation canal, the High Line brought water to some 20,000 acres along its 71-mile length.

When it was completed in 1883, the canal was a straightforward commercial venture: It brought drinking water to settlers and irrigation water to farmers out on the dry prairie. But over the next hundred years, the somewhat leaky canal created an emerald strand of vegetation through the metro Denver area. The canal's water nurtured lawns, trees, gardens, and golf courses. In fact, the canal has spawned a micro-ecosystem of its own along most of its 71-mile length, from the Dakota Hogback to far out in the open, arid prairie.

Water flows in the canal from April through October, although not always continuously. In winter runoff from storms and snowmelt fills its bed.

Today Denver Water Department, the regional water utility, owns and controls the water in the canal, although there are still some one hundred landowners with rights to the water flow. The High Line Canal Trail is the responsibility of a number of metropolitan entities.

Starting at the south end, the trail is under Chatfield Park jurisdiction from Waterton Canyon to Plum Creek. Highlands Ranch Metropolitan District oversees the portion from Santa Fe Drive to County Line Road.

In Arapahoe County, the stretch from County Line Road to Hampden Avenue is a model of maintenance and thoughtful provision of amenities for hikers. The South Suburban Recreation District, which has overseen this portion since 1970, has installed numerous benches and refuse receptacles; it also keeps the banks mowed so that access to water is plentiful.

The Denver Parks and Recreation Department administers the portion from Eisenhower Park to Havana Street near the Cherry Creek Dam and a strip through the Green Valley Ranch area. The canal trail is for the most part paved in Denver, although there are stretches of hard-packed dirt.

Finally, from Havana Street to I–70 the canal trail falls under the jurisdiction of the Aurora Parks and Open Space Department. The trail is paved in parts, while farther east it's mostly dirt packed. Here out in the prairie, the canal is a mere shadow of its robust self farther south—it's just a narrow ditch with only intermittent water.

The High Line Canal Trail is a flat path covered with dirt, crushed granite, or pavement the width of a narrow lane; it's open to hikers, bikers, and horses. Although popular on weekends, it makes for a quiet, riparian retreat from the urban and suburban sprawl through

3

which it meanders. In many years the lush greenery along the canal's banks creates a welcome respite on a hot summer day. In spring wild asparagus grows in infrequent clumps on the banks, which are lined with hundred-year-old cottonwoods, willows, wild plums, and chokecherries, the vegetation providing shelter for ducks, Canada geese, foxes, raccoons, and, more recently, coyotes.

Today more than half a million people annually use the canal trail, which has been designated a National Landmark Trail. Surveys show that 199 species of birds, fifteen reptiles, and twenty-eight mammals make their home along the canal's banks.

The trail is a flat, easy walk that drops only 2 feet per mile. Sturdy shoes are a good idea, however, as is keeping a keen eye on your dog's progress. Sharp, nasty thorns called goat heads scatter along the edges of the trail during fall and winter; they can get stuck between the pads of your companion's paws, and sometimes even penetrate a thin sole.

Brown mile markers posted on the mountain side of the canal mark distances along the canal trail. South Suburban Recreation District has added its own markers, which are in the shape of a stylized S.

The High Line Canal Trail doesn't take you quickly from here to there. Rather, it follows the canal along its loops and oxbows. Think of it as a leisurely stroll savored for the pleasure of the journey.

South Platte River Greenway

The South Platte River begins as runoff on the Continental Divide near Fairplay, an old mining town in South Park, some 60 miles west of Denver. After joining the North Platte, the river flows through Nebraska to Missouri. The Platte is a wide, slow-moving river on the High Plains—hence its name, which is French for "flat." (It was named by French fur trappers in the mid-1850s.)

As it exits the Front Range southwest of Denver, the South Platte winds through four counties and eight municipalities. The river passes dozens of municipal parks, nature preserves, and a mosaic of urban and suburban landscapes. With the exception of Chatfield

State Park, the greenway trail follows the rivercourse.

The Platte was the route that North American fur traders, early explorers, and settlers followed on their journey westward. Now a shared-use recreational trail, the South Platte River Greenway is the spine of Denver's trail system. Not only does the river flow through the heart of the city, but it's also the waterway that all other creeks in the area eventually empty into, with the exception of the man-made High Line Canal.

The South Platte River Greenway came into being in the environmentally conscious 1970s. Walking the well-landscaped and attractive trail, it's difficult to remember that the South Platte was a wasteland prior to Earth Day 1970, the first Earth Day. In 1974 Bill McNichols, then Denver's mayor, named the Platte River Development Committee and transferred for its use $1.9 million in federal revenue-sharing funds. The committee eventually became the Platte River Greenway Foundation, which raised some $15 million to build paths, bridges, parks, and boat ramps as well as undertake a massive river cleanup.

The Platte River Greenway was arguably the first project that applied the term *greenway* to a major urban trail and resource preservation corridor. It helped spawn an international greenway movement that resulted in more than 500 greenway projects across the United States and Canada.

Restoration of the Platte within the Denver city limits was completed in 1984. The cleanup subsequently expanded north and south. Arapahoe County's 8 miles of paths were completed in the 1980s at a cost of $4 million. Nine miles in Adams County were finished in 1996 at a cost of $2.5 million. Restoration efforts are ongoing along the Platte: Adams County has plans to extend the greenbelt eventually to the city of Brighton, where a portion has already been funded by income earmarked from the Colorado Lottery.

Meanwhile, in Denver, an additional $45 million in funds has created a new thirty-acre green space, the largest park to be constructed in Denver in the twentieth century, in Central Platte

Valley, the area between LoDo and I–25.

Efforts to restore the South Platte have been rewarded with the return of many bird species, including the great blue heron, a large and majestic bird that can be spotted perched on rocks in midstream. The river helps filter water while providing valuable food and cover to animals such as muskrats, foxes, and raccoons. For the walker, the river environment provides solace, recreation, and a lasting feeling of peace.

In Denver and in Adams County, the greenway trail is paved and is a favorite excursion route for bicyclists and in-line skaters. Thus, large stretches of the greenway trail are not suited for a walker with a dog: The pavement narrows in places to only 8 feet across. Since the greenway path also hugs a road in many instances, your ability to maneuver a pet on a leash is further diminished.

In Denver, eleven parks create buffers between the river and urban noise and activity. During the river restoration process, the waterway was cleared and dredged with a deep channel that eliminates springtime flooding. From May through September, the river's constant water flow makes kayaking and rafting possible, with one launching ramp just blocks away from Coors Field in lower downtown (LoDo).

Perhaps because of the deepening of the channel, the banks of the Platte tend to be steep in Denver. Also, rapids were put in place to minimize erosion; these create strong currents in many places. The banks are thickly overgrown with brush, so your pet's access to the water is limited.

Beyond the greenbelt itself, industrial activity is ongoing. Portions of the greenway pass not only manufacturing plants, such as the Robinson Brick Company, but also garbage depots and car junkyards.

For these reasons, I've selected walks along the Platte River Greenway that run along a park or are located at the junction with one of the river's many tributaries, where there's more open space and access to water.

Mileage markers along the greenway vary from jurisdiction to jurisdiction, as does the greenway's name. In Denver it's called the Platte River and Cherry Creek Greenway, while in Arapahoe County it's the Platte River Greenway. In Littleton it's called the Carson Greenway, in honor of Mary Carson, former chair of the South Suburban Park Foundation, which, during her tenure, spearheaded the extension of the greenway south past the Denver city limits.

The most consistent signage is in Arapahoe County. Distances between major access points along the trail are given on plaques, while mileage is etched in red on brown posts. In Chatfield State Park there are no directional signs or mileage markers for the greenway trail.

Cherry Creek Greenway

Cherry Creek flows into the South Platte at Confluence Park in the shadow of Coors Field, the home of the Colorado Rockies. Like the Platte River, Cherry Creek has been tied closely with the history and growth of Denver. Gold was discovered in the creek in 1858, and the discovery made Denver a boomtown. As the town grew, spring floods along the creek became an annual menace, but it was not until 1950 that the creek was harnessed by the Cherry Creek Dam, built by the U.S. Army Corp of Engineers, south of Denver in Aurora. The resulting reservoir and surrounding state park are popular for boating, swimming, hiking, biking, and camping. The corridor along the creek was reclaimed in the 1970s and 1980s for recreation by the same Platte River Greenway Foundation that revitalized the South Platte. The Cherry Creek bike path and adjoining trails connect the South Platte with Cherry Creek State Park and the High Line Canal Trail system.

The greenway runs through the heart of the Denver metro area. It touches the center city and is paved for its entire length. Although a favorite of bikers and in-line skaters, the greenbelt is wide enough in many places to provide an adjacent dirt trail, preferred by hikers. In addition, several parks that run alongside the greenway offer extra room for a dog on a leash.

Access remains the most problematic part about walking with

your dog along the Cherry Creek Greenway. From Larimer Street to University Boulevard, the greenbelt runs between the north- and southbound lanes of Speer Boulevard, which necessitates crossing a very busy street. For this reason, the center-city walk selected for this book was chosen because it includes a pedestrian cross signal.

From Confluence Park to Colfax Avenue, there are two concrete paths. The bike path, which is also used by skaters, runs along the west bank of the creek to Colfax Avenue; the east-bank path is restricted to pedestrian traffic.

From Colfax Avenue to Downing Street, the creek is channeled between banks that have been landscaped with a terrace of boulders. The banks are covered with grass that is regularly cut, and there are many places where you can step off the paved trail to give your dog access to the water.

The creek is closed to pedestrian traffic in the portion that passes through the Denver Country Club, which is private. East of University Boulevard the creek trail runs alongside the Cherry Creek Shopping Center, another section that's beautifully landscaped and maintained.

East of Colorado Boulevard the creek passes through Glendale, a small city surrounded by Denver.

From Monaco Boulevard east to its intersection with the High Line Canal near Yosemite Street, the greenway runs along Cherry Creek Drive; it's narrow here, and not particularly hospitable to walkers or their dogs. East of the intersection with the High Line, the creek trail passes through a large open meadow, which offers numerous side dirt trails as well as easy water access.

On the east side of Havana, the creek trail is essentially a narrow access path that climbs up to the Cherry Creek Dam before descending to the park. Inside the park the trail runs for a significant section along a wetland area where pets are not permitted. The trail then emerges onto and crosses the dog training area (see Walk 40) in the southeastern portion of the park.

Sand Creek Regional Greenway

Denver's newest greenway is the Sand Creek Regional Greenway. Sand Creek originates in southeast Aurora, intersects the High Line Canal, and flows north for 13 miles through portions of Denver and Commerce City, where it empties into the South Platte River and connects with the Platte River Greenway.

The high plains flanking Sand Creek were the scene of settlements and encampments by Native American tribes as well as their buffalo hunting grounds. Early settlers established wagon routes that crisscrossed this wide prairie and the stream. Later these routes became stagecoach stops and, later still, railroad rights-of-way that cut off the creek from recreational use. Industrial development and warehousing followed the railroad to the creek, and the natural habitat of the area was severely degraded. Today Sand Creek runs through one of Colorado's most heavily urbanized and human-impacted areas.

For the past fifty years, only 6 miles of Sand Creek have been open to recreation. Following the closing of Stapleton International Airport in 1995, another 3-mile stretch became available for redevelopment. The creation of continuous access to the creek has led to a joint venture by Aurora, Denver, and Commerce City to develop a unified recreational plan for Sand Creek corridor.

Sand Creek today is lined with cottonwoods, willows, and open stretches of prairie. Although some parts of the creek have been marred by indiscriminate dumping, which has polluted the water and created eyesores, recent surveys have shown that the creek is home to significant wildlife populations, including deer, foxes, beavers, herons, owls, and egrets. The creation of the Sand Creek Regional Greenway initiated the ongoing revitalization of the habitat along the creek through an influx of funds from two successful lawsuits brought by the Sierra Club and the involvement of northeast metro youth and community groups in the restoration. Eventually a continuous trail will link historic and environmentally significant sites along Sand Creek.

The cooperative effort is not only repairing damaged areas but also bringing jogging, biking, and hiking opportunities to the eastern metro area. The completion of the Sand Creek Regional Greenway will make it possible to hike and bike around the entire metro area on linked riverside trails.

Sand Creek is clearly still a greenbelt in the making, but its potential, as you'll see from the two walks described in this guide, is tremendous. The trails along the creek range from overgrown jeep roads to a new crushed-aggregate surface to pavement. The banks of Sand Creek slope gently in the area of these two walks, and your pet will have many opportunities to take a quick dip at the water's edge.

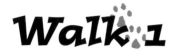

Walk 1

Platte Canyon Reservoir

General location: Waterton Canyon in the southwest metro area.

Special attractions: Scenic vistas, solitude, and a bucolic landscape.

Open: 5 A.M. to 10 P.M.

Total distance: 4 miles round trip; 2 miles as a shuttle.

Estimated time: 1 ½ to 2 hours.

Services: None.

Restrictions: Keep your dog on a leash. Watch out for free-roaming cattle alongside the canal.

For more information: Chatfield State Park, (303) 791–7275.

Getting started

From C–470 take the Wadsworth Boulevard (C–121) exit south and continue on South Wadsworth Boulevard for 4.8 miles to a clearly marked turnoff for Waterton Canyon. Turn left (east) onto Waterton Road and continue for 0.3 mile, past the trail entrance and parking lot for the Colorado Trail/Waterton Canyon Trail. Cross a bridge over the South Platte River. Look for a large rock outcropping on your right. Park on the wide shoulder of the road; there's room for three cars. The entrance to the High Line Canal trail is across the road. In summer the sign may be obscured by tall grass. There's also a dirt parking lot a few hundred feet down the road on your left; its entrance can also be obscured by grass in summer.

If you want to do this walk as a shuttle with a friend, continue on Waterton Road to its end at Rampart Range Road (County Road 5). Turn left (east) and drive for 1.2 miles to pulloffs on either side of the road at a small bridge over the High Line Canal. A yellow sign warns about a school bus stop several hundred feet ahead. Leave

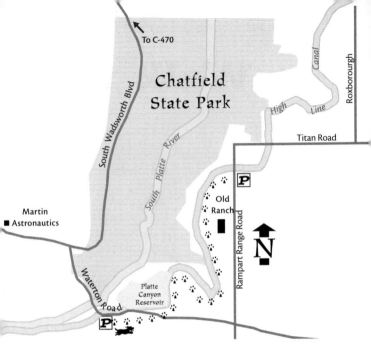

one of your cars here and return in the other to the High Line Canal access near the South Platte River.

Overview

If you're looking for solitude, great views, bird life, and a glimpse of what this area looked like at the beginning of the twentieth century, you'll find them here. The canal begins nearly 2 miles up the canyon to the west. A diversion dam on the South Platte River funnels water into a 600-foot-long tunnel. Water is siphoned beneath the river and carried in flumes around several gulches as it flows toward Waterton Road. South of Waterton Road the canal flows through private property; a closed gate bars access.

Once across the road, the canal passes through the southeast corner of Chatfield State Park, then through a private ranch where an original, tin-roofed homesteader's log cabin is still in use. Since the ranch owns land on both sides of the canal, you may encounter cattle on the canal trail or see animals in the pasture along the banks.

Take note of your surroundings: This is one of the last fragments of tallgrass prairie along the Front Range. Distant stands of native scrub oak and thick willow groves near the water provide wildlife habitat and shelter for deer, foxes, skunks, coyotes, rabbits, and numerous raptors, including eagles.

The walk

🐾 If you parked on the shoulder of Waterton Road, leash your dog and cross the road. If you parked in the lot, walk down the edge of the road to the canal trail on the north side of the road. Turn right onto the trail. Almost immediately you'll see a large HIGH LINE CANAL sign on your left.

🐾 Continue on the canal trail past the Platte Canyon Reservoir to the north. The reservoir stores water from the High Line Canal for late release into the South Platte River. A high chain-link fence surrounds it.

The two white clapboard buildings are pumping sheds. Stop at the second shed to read a sign from a gentler age. Instead of the present day's brusque KEEP OUT, this rusted sign advises, COMMIT NO NUISANCE HERE. THESE WATERS ARE PUBLIC WATER SUPPLY. THE DEFILEMENT OF THESE WATERS IN ANY WAY IS STRICTLY NOT ALLOWED.

🐾 Pass mile marker 2 on your left and continue to the first wire gate across the trail. Use the side wooden gate to continue. The canal sweeps in a large lazy loop, creating a low pasture that's fed by Little Willow Creek.

The giant cottonwoods in this area date back to the canal's construction in the 1880s. Some of the tree trunks have a circumference that exceeds three arm spans. In the distance to the northeast, Denver's skyline is visible. Keep a close watch on your pet here: A herd of cattle may be grazing on the edge of the canal or resting in the shade of the cottonwoods.

🦴 Pass a homesteader's log cabin on the opposite bank of the canal, then continue to the second wire gate. Pass through the small wooden gate on your right.

🦴 Continue to a third gate just short of Rampart Range Road. A horse farm is on your left. At the canal crossing over the road, turn around and return the way you came, or retrieve one of your cars if your walk was a shuttle.

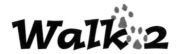

Walk 2

Highlands Ranch

General location: Highlands
Ranch in Douglas County.

Special attractions:
Spectacular views of the
Front Range and the Denver
skyline.

Open: 5 A.M. to 10 P.M.

Total distance: 3.8 miles round
trip if you start at Town
Center Road.

Estimated time: 2 hours.

Services: Numerous services,
including rest rooms at
Redstone Park.

Restrictions: Your dog must be
on a leash.

For more information:
Highlands Ranch
Metropolitan Districts
(303) 791–2710.

Getting started

Although Highlands Ranch's development began in the late 1980s,
until recently the portion of the High Line Canal that flows through
the huge development's western segments had been difficult for
residents to access. The opening of Redstone Park in 2000 changed
that. The park is located across the street from a ramp built in
1999 that provides access to the High Line Canal Trail. The ramp
skirts the Highlands Ranch Golf Club, which straddles the canal,
and accesses the canal trail by means of a bridge that's also used by
golfers. There's plentiful parking at two lots in Redstone Park.

To reach Redstone Park from C–470, take the Lucent Boulevard
exit and go south on Lucent Boulevard for 0.6 mile to its intersection
with Town Center Drive. Turn right (west) onto Town Center Drive
and continue for 0.8 mile to Redstone Park on the left (south)
side of the street. You can either park in a lot off Foothills Canyon
Boulevard or continue to the main lot in the center of the park. A
dog run is across the street, on the east side of Foothills Canyon
Boulevard (see Walk 42.)

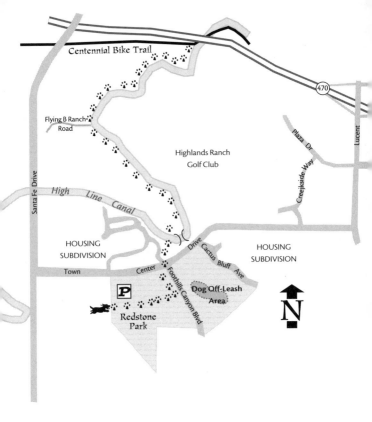

Overview

Perhaps the finest views of the Front Range and of Denver's skyline along the High Line can be seen in this area, where the canal makes a large lazy loop to the east after it crosses Santa Fe Drive. A private ranch located adjacent to the Highlands Ranch Golf Club provides unobstructed views to the west and north. Look for golden eagles on the branches of the tall cottonwoods. Native prairie plants along this stretch include blue grama, tall fescue, and western wheat grass.

Highlands Ranch draws water from the canal through a headgate in this area.

The walk

〇══〇 Park your vehicle and leash your dog. If you parked in the middle of Redstone Park, walk east (left) past a pavilion, a small pond, and a second pavilion to Foothills Canyon Boulevard and turn left. Cross Town Center Drive. Once across the road look for a concrete ramp leading down to the canal. Cross the bridge to the canal trail. Watch out for golf carts.

Stately cottonwoods form a shaded glade here. As the canal turns north and west, the panorama of mountains opens to your left. Before you lie undulating pastures and hillsides. Longs Peak is visible to the northwest, while Mount Evans rises to the west, beyond the hogback and the foothills. The banks of the canal are not steep in this area, although grassy slopes alternate with stands of willows. In between the cottonwoods, Denver's skyline shimmers in the haze like the castle in *The Wizard of Oz*.

〇══〇 At 1 mile a private drive to the left leads to the Flying B Ranch, whose pastures spread to the west. The canal leaves the bend and continues in a northerly direction. A little farther on McLellan Reservoir, which holds some canal water, creates an awesome foreground to the panorama of mountains to the north and west.

〇══〇 At 1.4 miles the canal intersects with the Centennial Bicycle Trail, which follows C–470 and South Wadsworth Boulevard to Waterton Canyon. Turn around and return the way you came.

〇══〇 The next 2.2 miles of the canal trail are concrete and very popular with bicyclists.

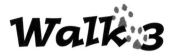

Walk 3

Writer Vista Park

General location: Littleton.

Special attractions: Scenic vistas with several benches on which to sit and enjoy them. Five local parks are adjacent to the canal, and there's easy access to swimming for your pet from the grassy, gentle canal bank.

Open: 6 A.M. to 11 P.M.

Total distance: 5 miles round trip.

Estimated time: 2 to 2½ hours.

Services: Rest rooms, water, picnic tables.

Restrictions: Your dog must be on a leash no longer than 6 feet.

For more information: South Suburban Park and Recreation District, (303) 789–5131.

Getting started

From Santa Fe Drive, take Mineral Avenue east for 1 mile to its intersection with Peninsula Drive. Turn right (south). The parking lot is immediately on your left. There is a pedestrian crossover signal at Mineral Avenue.

Overview

This is a shaded, pleasant walk on a greenbelt bordered by rural, horse properties on the west and more recent subdivisions on the east side of the canal. When the canal passes one of the five parks along the trail, the landscape opens up on distant views of the Front Range. Some benches along the way are placed in the shade, while others are located at strategic points that offer panoramic vistas. The banks of the canal are grassy and well maintained amid stands of thick willows that grow where shade is scant. There are numerous

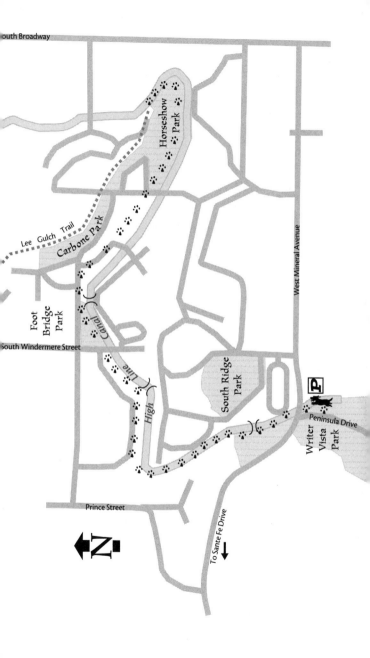

South Broadway

Horseshow Park

Lee Gulch Trail

Carbone Park

West Mineral Avenue

Foot
Bridge
Park

South Windermere Street

Canal Line

South Ridge Park

High

Writer Vista Park

Peninsula Drive

Prince Street

To Sante Fe Drive

N

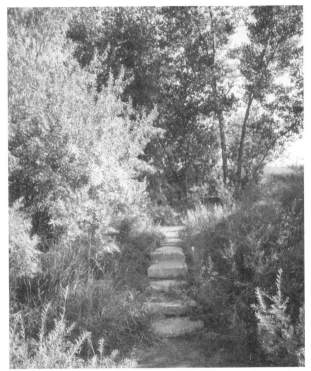

A shaded path leads from the High Line Canal to a nearby tennis court at Writer Vista Park.

points where you can lead your pet to the water for a dip.

The walk

🦴 Writer Vista Park is the gateway to this hike. Rest rooms and picnic tables are found in the southwest corner of the park, across Peninsula Drive. Like other portions of the High Line Canal Trail, this stretch can be accessed from several starting points, but the parking lot at Writer Vista Park is most convenient.

🦴 After parking your vehicle and putting a leash (no longer than 6 feet) on your dog, cross Mineral Avenue at the crosswalk that has a signal. The crushed-aggregate trail meanders through rural Littleton. Soon a bridge leads to a private tennis club. Look for bird- and bat houses mounted in the cottonwoods.

In the distance the V-shaped cut you see in the Dakota Hogback is the gateway to the Ken Caryl Ranch development. The fruit trees on the west side of the canal are Newport plums.

🦴 At 0.7 mile the trail passes through the original part of Littleton, which remains semirural. At 1 mile another bridge leads to Dry Creek Road. Be careful at the crossing of South Windermere Street, shortly after. Cross another bridge at 1.2 miles at Footbridge Park. Mature trees shade the homes here, while conifers create privacy barriers as well as shelter for wildlife.

🦴 Cross Gallup Street, a quiet local street, at 1.4 mile, then Horseshoe Park. Turn around when you reach the intersection with the Lee Gulch Trail (2 miles); this trail heads west to the South Platte River Greenway. On your right a flume across the drainage carries the canal water. At this point the canal trail veers to the left for about 150 feet before regaining the canal bank. Return the way you came.

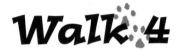

Walk 4

DeKoevend Open Space Park

General location: Littleton.

Special attractions: Views of the Front Range, a parklike setting, an exercise area, and a playground.

Open: 6 A.M. to 11 P.M.

Total distance: 4.8 miles round trip.

Estimated time: 2 to 2½ hours.

Services: Rest rooms, water fountains, telephones in the recreational center.

Restrictions: Your dog must be on a leash no longer than 6 feet.

For more information: South Suburban Park and Recreation District, (303) 789–5131.

Getting started

Getting to this section of South University Boulevard from a major highway isn't easy, because the street runs through the center of the metro area and isn't near any of the interstates in this area. One way to access this walk is to take exit 201 (Hampden Avenue) heading west from I–25. Continue for 2 miles to the intersection with University Boulevard. Turn left (south) and drive 3.7 miles to the intersection with Orchard Road. Go through the intersection and stay in the right lane. As University Boulevard bends around the High Line Canal, look for a large parking lot on the west side of the street and a sign that says JULIA DEKOEVEND PARK. Pull into the lot. Park on the west side of the lot, near the bridge that leads over the canal.

Overview

DeKoevend Open Space Park occupies land in a large bend of the High Line Canal and offers a variety of amenities, ranging from

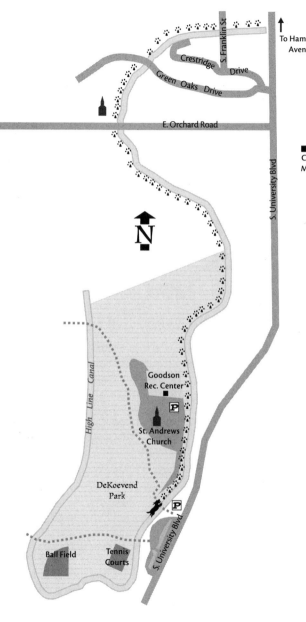

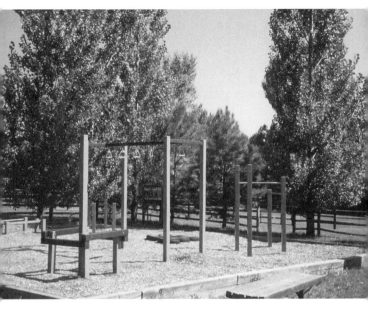

This outdoor exercise area at DeKoevend Open Space Park contains seven different exercise options, including chinning bars and a squat stretch.

covered picnic areas to rest rooms, as well as access to the Goodson Recreation Center and its full complement of sports activities and facilities. Numerous trails and several bridges crisscross the park. A variety of excursions are possible.

The walk described here begins in the park, passes the recreation center, and accesses an exercise area and playground that are unique along the canal trail. The exercise area is north of the recreation center.

The banks of the canal here are grassy and offer numerous places where your pet can access the water.

Walk 4 / DeKoevend Open Space Park

The walk

🦴After parking your vehicle and leashing your dog (the leash cannot be longer than 6 feet), cross the canal on a bridge on the west side of the parking lot and turn right (north). You'll immediately come upon several playing fields of the South Suburban Recreation Park and District as well as rest rooms, water fountain, and covered picnic tables. Continue for 0.2 mile to the Goodson Recreation Center, operated by South Suburban Park and Recreation District.

Immediately after you pass the recreation center, the trees and the land falls away and a panoramic view of the Rocky Mountains opens before you. Eagles and great horned owls frequent this area.

🦴Be careful crossing Orchard Road; there's no pedestrian signal. On the north side of Orchard, the Church of Latter Day Saints has built a children's playground that's open to canal hikers. In addition to a slide and swings, you'll find a bench in the shade where an adult can rest and admire the nearby bed of annual flowers.

Notice the outdoor exercise area located between Green Oaks Drive and Franklin Street. This well-equipped station contains seven different exercise options, including chinning bars, a vertical ladder, parallel bars, a squat stretch, and more. Signs at each location give instructions on how to use the equipment. There's also a sign that instructs you on how to check your pulse.

The canal bank is steep in spots, but there are also several opportunities for your pet to get to the water.

🦴Turn around at the underpass at University Boulevard. Built in 1999 by Greenwood Village, this underpass eliminates a dangerous surface crossing. Return the way you came.

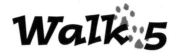

Walk 5

Orchard Road to Long Road

General location: Greenwood Village.

Special attractions: A shaded path, easy access to water, and a nice setting.

Open: 6 A.M. to 11 P.M.

Total distance: 3 miles round trip (3.5 miles with a short side trip for refreshments at Cherry Hills Marketplace, at Orchard Road and University Boulevard).

Estimated time: 1 to 1½ hours.

Services: Portable toilets in the parking lot.

Restrictions: Your dog must be on a leash no longer than 6 feet.

For more information: South Suburban Park and Recreation District, (303) 789–5131.

Getting started

Take exit 198 (Orchard Road) off I-25 and drive west for 2.5 miles to the gravel parking lot on the north side of the road where it crosses the canal. This lot holds thirty or so cars.

Overview

With the installation of a good-sized parking lot where the High Line Canal crosses Orchard Road in Greenwood Village, the canal trail stretching both north and south has increased in popularity and use. The 1.46-mile section between Orchard Road and Long Road passes the confluence of the High Line Canal with Little Dry Creek, then continues in a northwesterly direction under the shade of hundred-year-old cottonwoods. An interesting landmark is a small tree nursery.

Like other portions of the High Line Canal Trail, this stretch can be walked from several starting points, but the parking lot at Orchard Road offers the easiest access.

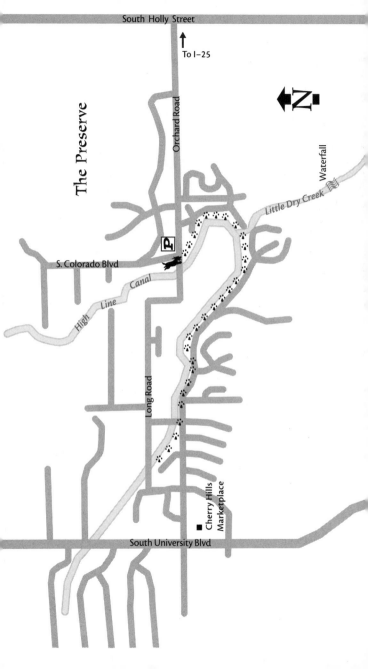

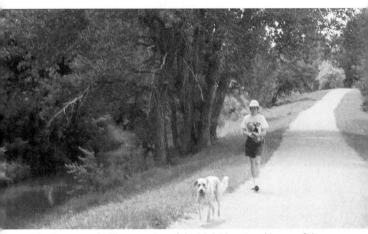

The Greenwood Village portion of the High Line Canal is one of the most popular with dog owners.

The walk

🦴 After parking your vehicle and leashing your dog (the leash cannot be longer than 6 feet), cross the pedestrian portion of the small bridge over the canal, then cross Orchard Road. Watch out for traffic, because there's no pedestrian crosswalk signal. Begin your walk on the hard-packed dirt trail. On your right you'll pass the Little Dry Creek District office of the Denver Water Department. As soon as the chain-link fence ends (about 100 yards), make a sharp turn right and proceed on a trail through the water department's maintenance yard.

🦴 Look for a small white sign on the canal trail that indicates with an arrow the trail cut through the water department's property. If the yard is closed, a sign directs you to an alternate path along a neighborhood trail. The canal itself loops around to the north and west. A siphon carries the canal water under the intersecting Little Dry Creek. If you stay to the left, you'll find yourself on the Little Dry Creek Trail and near a waterfall, which

28

means you've strayed from the High Line Canal.

Back on the canal trail, you'll pass a tree nursery on your right established by the Denver Water Department and South Suburban Park and Recreation District. Thus far the nursery has provided more than 300 trees to replace aging cottonwoods along the canal.

🐾 The canal trail now passes under stately cottonwoods that block out the heat of the day. The next mile offers a quiet, country club atmosphere. The bank is gently sloped in several places, and your dog can take a quick dip. Continue on to where the canal crosses Long Road.

🐾 Your option here is to return the way you came or make a 0.3-mile detour to the Cherry Hills Marketplace for refreshments. If you chose the side trip, turn left (west) onto the sidewalk along Long Road and walk a short block to the intersection of Long Road and Long Lane. At the stop sign turn left (south) and proceed for another block. Long Lane ends at Orchard Road. (This is the same Orchard Road that you used to get to the parking lot where you left your car. The eastern segment of this road doesn't connect with the western, however, because of the confluence of the High Line Canal and Little Dry Creek and the siphons and flumes you passed earlier on this walk.) Once you're on Orchard Road, turn right (west) and cross the road: You're in the Cherry Hills Marketplace. Alfalfa's, the health food store, has a small restaurant that in good weather offers seating at metal tables outside the store. Bistro-type tables are also arranged in front of a Starbucks coffee shop nearby.

You can also extend your walk at the point where the canal trail crosses Long Road. The canal trail continues for just under 0.5 mile through horse pastures to University Boulevard. Here a wide, well-lit underpass takes hikers safely under the boulevard. The underpass was completed in 1999 to eliminate a dangerous surface crossing. Greenwood Village was instrumental in getting the underpass built and funded the construction.

🐾 When you're ready, turn around and return the way you came.

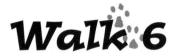

Walk 6

Orchard Road to Belleview Avenue

General location: Greenwood
Village.

Special attractions: Rural
atmosphere; panoramic views
of the Front Range; sightings
of foxes, eagles, and deer.
There are occasional benches
along the route.

Open: 6 A.M. to 11 P.M.

Total distance: 5.8 miles round
trip, although returning on
a portion of the Greenwood

Village Equestrian Trail cuts
off about a mile.

Estimated time: 2 to 3 hours.

Services: Portable toilets are in
the parking lot.

Restrictions: Your dog must be
on a leash no longer than 6
feet.

For more information: South
Suburban Park and
Recreation District,
(303) 789–5131.

Getting started

Take exit 198 (Orchard Road) from I–25 and drive west for 2.5 miles
to the gravel parking lot on the north side of the road where it
crosses the canal. The lot holds thirty or so cars.

Overview

With the installation of a good-sized parking lot where the High
Line Canal crosses Orchard Road in Greenwood Village, the canal
trail stretching both north and south has increased in popularity
and use. This 2.9-mile section between Orchard Road and Belleview
Avenue—and particularly the 1-mile portion between Orchard
Road and Williamette Lane—offers views of the Front Range that
take your breath away no matter how many times you've seen
the vista.

The sparsely built character of the Orchard-Williamette area,

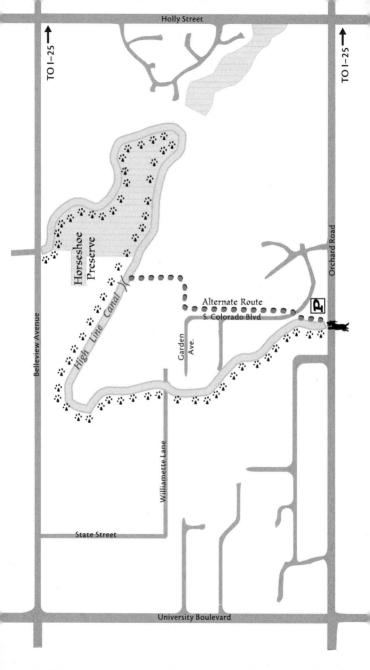

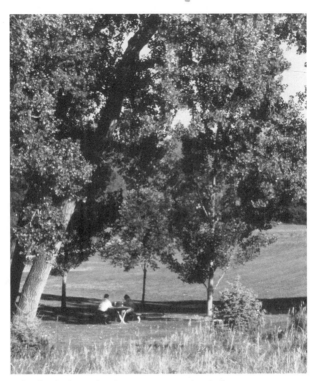

A family picnics under the trees on a weekend afternoon.

which is known as rural Greenwood and was once a farming community, enhances the feeling of openness. The zoning here divides the land into parcels ranging from two and a half acres up to ten or more, and there are still several small working farms. One of these, on Long Road due west of the canal, produces a bumper crop of pumpkins that are offered for sale every October.

The walk

Although this stretch can be walked from several starting points (including other portions of the High Line Canal Trail), the Orchard

Road parking lot offers the easiest access.

🐾 After parking your vehicle and leashing your dog (the leash cannot be longer than 6 feet), cross the canal on the pedestrian portion of the small bridge and turn right (north) onto the hard-packed dirt trail.

The highlights of this walk become immediately apparent. Panoramic views to the west sweep from Mount Evans to Longs Peak. Pass an old red barn on the opposite bank that harks back to early settlers. Sightings of hawks, ducks, Canada geese, foxes, deer, and even coyotes are common in this area. The trail offers numerous gentle descents to the canal, where your dog can put his feet in.

Since the trail serves as a levee, you are always slightly higher than the sloping land to the west and therefore can enjoy the panoramic views of the Front Range for most of the walk. The Orchard-Williamette portion is uncommonly quiet, bucolic, and rural, since there are no through streets here.

🐾 Just before you reach Williamette Lane, there's a bench where you can sit down to rest or enjoy the view. At 1 mile the canal trail crosses Williamette Lane, a narrow, rural street that provides restricted access to a horse farm and another home on the east side of the canal, where the lane dead-ends. Past Williamette there are two horse farms on the west side of the canal as well as several houses as the canal bends toward Belleview Avenue.

🐾 In the next 0.25 mile, Belleview Avenue traffic noise intrudes on the silence, but the trail and canal veer to the southeast to form a 1.5-mile-long, sweeping curve around a wildlife preserve and park owned by Greenwood Village. Two benches in this area offer prime places to sit quietly and sight birds and other wildlife.

🐾 At the start of the curve, look across the canal: A double row of split-rail fencing marks a partially complete equestrian trail on the east side of the canal. A few hundred feet past mile marker South Suburban 6.5, an equestrian bridge crosses the canal and leads to the Greenwood Village trail system.

Beyond the equestrian bridge, the canal trail loops back west then north and passes a subdivision of luxury town homes on the east side of the canal.

🦴 Turn around at the underpass at Belleview Avenue and return the way you came.

Alternate route

For a different way back, cross the canal at the equestrian bridge. Immediately turn right (south) and follow the dirt road for about 0.25 mile until it ends in the aggregate-improved equestrian trail mentioned earlier. The trail turns east, then south, then west around three houses. It emerges at the intersection of Garden Avenue where South Colorado Boulevard dead-ends. The trail follows the east side of Colorado Boulevard for 0.5 mile, then crosses it where the street touches the east bank of the High Line Canal. The trail continues for a few hundred feet along the east side of the canal before emerging at the north end of the parking lot at Orchard Road.

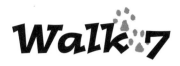

Walk 7

Dahlia Street to Belleview Avenue

General location: Cherry Hills Village.

Special attractions: Scenic views of the Front Range, large homes, open space, and several ponds.

Open: 6 A.M. to 11 P.M.

Total distance: 3.3 miles round trip.

Estimated time: 1 to 1½ hours.

Services: None.

Restrictions: Your dog must be kept on a leash no longer than 6 feet.

For more information: South Suburban Park and Recreation District, (303) 789–5131.

Getting started

Take exit 204 (Colorado Boulevard) off I–25. Turn south (right) onto Colorado Boulevard and drive 3 miles to Quincy Street. Turn left (east) onto Quincy and drive 0.3 mile to a stop sign at Dahlia Street. Turn right (south) and drive 3 blocks to the end of the road and the parking lot on the High Line Canal.

Overview

The large grounds of the Kent Denver Day School were originally assembled in the 1950s for a possible retirement home for President Dwight D. Eisenhower and his wife, Mamie, who was born and grew up in Denver. The plans never came to fruition, though, because the Eisenhowers retired to a farm in Gettysburg, Pennsylvania. Today the acreage is occupied by a private school.

The walk

After parking your vehicle and leashing your dog (the leash cannot be longer than 6 feet), begin by crossing the wooden bridge

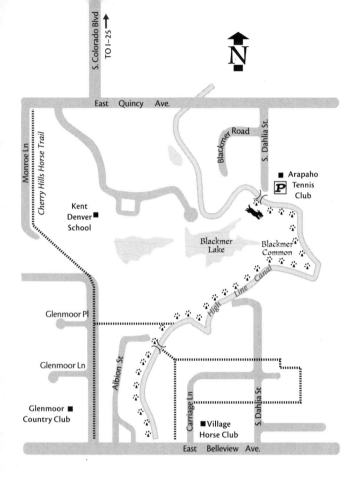

over the canal. Turn left (south) and walk for 1.65 miles to the underpass at Belleview Avenue. The trip offers panoramic vistas of the Front Range.

Blackmer Common at 0.6 mile was donated and designated as open space. You may walk into this fifteen-acre preserve. The area is adjacent to the private Kent Denver Day School. Bald eagles, coyotes, and foxes have been spotted here, because the wetlands are a favorite wintering location for large flocks of Canada geese.

🦴 An unimproved horse trail bearing to the west skirts the Glenmoor Country Club and heads north to East Quincy Avenue. The bridge at 1.5 miles leads to an undeveloped horse trail and open space open to the public.

🦴 At the Belleview Avenue underpass, turn around and return the way you came.

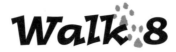

Walk 8

Dahlia Street to East Quincy Avenue

General location: Cherry Hills Village.

Special attractions: Scenic views of the Front Range, large homes, open space, and several ponds.

Open: 6 A.M. to 11 P.M.

Total distance: 1 mile round trip.

Estimated time: 30 to 40 minutes.

Services: None.

Restrictions: Your dog must be on a leash no longer than 6 feet.

For more information: South Suburban Park and Recreation District, (303) 789–5131.

Getting started

Take exit 204 (Colorado Boulevard) off I–25. Turn south (right) onto Colorado Boulevard and drive 3 miles to East Quincy Avenue. Turn left (east) onto Quincy and drive 0.3 miles to a stop sign at Dahlia Street. Turn right (south) and drive 3 blocks to the end of the road and the parking lot on the High Line Canal.

Overview

This is a quick, satisfying walk for those who wish to escape urban noise and congestion but have limited time. The trail also ranks high because of its lush vegetation, a small pond, and the feeling of peace and quiet that this area evokes. Although Cherry Hills is a desirable suburb, this stretch from Dahlia to Quincy has not been subjected to new construction for a number of years; the houses you glimpse through the mature vegetation are older.

The walk

After parking your vehicle and leashing your dog (the leash

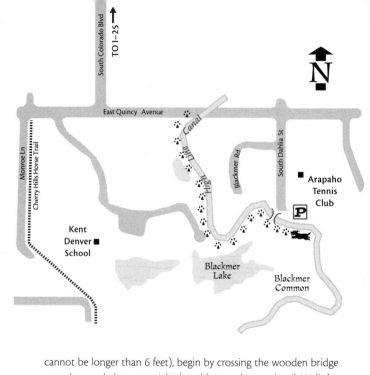

cannot be longer than 6 feet), begin by crossing the wooden bridge over the canal, then turn right (north) onto the canal trail. Walk for 0.5 mile to the spot where the canal crosses Quincy Avenue.

On your left is a private wildlife refuge with a pond and bird nesting boxes. Cherry Hills resident Catherine Anderson established this refuge. The canal trail is lined with tall shrubbery that narrows the trail to a country lane. A private bridge leads to a barn and corral where at one time there were several resident goats. I've also seen raccoons and foxes in this area.

🦴 At Quincy Avenue, turn around and return the way you came.

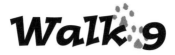

Walk 9

Colorado Boulevard to East Quincy Avenue

General location: Cherry Hills Village.

Special attractions: A pleasant park with horse-jumping equipment and weekend practices by a local pony club.

Open: 6 A.M. to 11 P.M.

Total distance: 1.6 miles round trip.

Estimated time: 30 minutes to 1 hour.

Services: None.

Restrictions: Your dog must be on a leash no longer than 6 feet.

For more information: South Suburban Park and Recreation District, (303) 789–5131.

Getting started

Take exit 204 (Colorado Boulevard) off I–25. Turn south (right) onto Colorado Boulevard and drive 2.7 miles. As you cross the small bridge over the High Line Canal, look for a small parking lot on your left. Three Pond Park, adjacent to the canal trail, has parking for about six cars.

Overview

Some of the loveliest stretches of the High Line Canal wind their leisurely way through Cherry Hills Village, where you can glimpse stone mansions, horse farms, and beautiful gardens from the canal trail. Only two small parking lots make this stretch of the canal accessible to nonresidents.

The walk

🦴 After parking your vehicle and leashing your dog (the leash cannot be longer than 6 feet), begin on the east side of Colorado

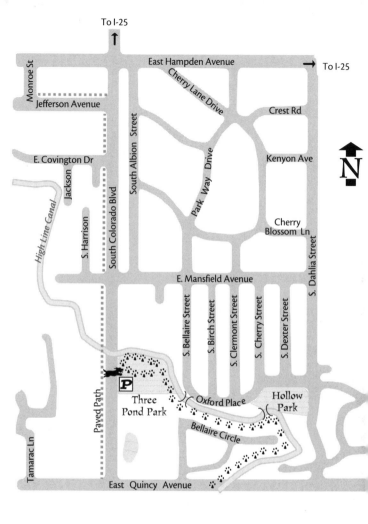

Boulevard and continue south on the canal trail for less than 100 yards. Leave the trail on a wide footpath that descends into Three Mile Park. A local pony club often uses the park for equestrian shows; there are wooden jumps on the broad meadow in the center of the small park. The footpath winds along the edge of the meadow, where several large logs serve as benches. The footpath crosses a small creek twice on a wooden bridge before rejoining the canal trail.

🦴 Continue south on the canal trail past two bridges over the canal that serve local residents. At East Quincy Avenue, turn around and return the way you came.

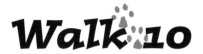

Walk 10

Colorado Boulevard to East Hampden Avenue

General location: Cherry Hills Village.

Special attractions: Large stately homes, a rural setting, and scenic views.

Open: 6 A.M. to 11 P.M.

Total distance: 2 miles round trip.

Estimated time: 40 minutes to 1 hour.

Services: None.

Restrictions: Your dog must be on a leash no longer than 6 feet.

For more information: South Suburban Park and Recreation District, (303) 789–5131.

Getting started

Take exit 204 (Colorado Boulevard) from I-25. Turn south onto Colorado Boulevard and drive 2.7 miles. As you cross the small bridge over the High Line Canal, look for a small parking lot on your left. Three Pond Park, adjacent to the canal trail, has parking for about six cars.

Overview

Some of the loveliest stretches of the High Line Canal wind their leisurely way through Cherry Hills Village, where you can glimpse mansions, horse farms, and manicured lawns from the canal trail. Only two small parking lots make this stretch of the canal accessible to nonresidents.

The walk

🦴After parking your vehicle, leash your dog and cross Colorado Boulevard to walk north on the canal trail. After the first bend in the

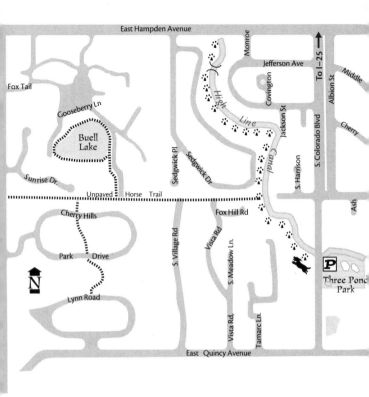

canal, an unimproved horse trail heads left (west). At 0.5 mile the canal trail meanders to the left, creating a grassy narrow meadow between the trail and the canal bank.

This is a good place to lead your pet down to the gently sloping bank for a refreshing dip in the canal. He can dry his coat by rolling in the thick grass, which receives regular mowing. Shortly before Hampden Avenue, a pedestrian bridge leads to local residences.

🦴 At Hampden Avenue, turn around and return the way you came. Although the canal flows under Hampden Avenue and through the Welshire Golf Course on the other side of the road, the canal trail is closed to the public.

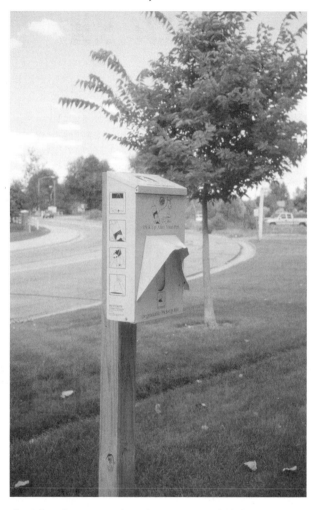

Plastic bag dispensers, such as this one, are available for dog owners in Denver Parks.

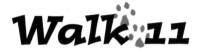

Walk 11

Eisenhower Park to I–25

General location: Southeast Denver.

Special attractions: A park with numerous facilities along a portion of the High Line Canal Trail.

Open: 6 A.M. to 11 P.M.

Total distance: 2 miles round trip.

Estimated time: 40 minutes to 1 hour.

Services: Rest rooms and water at the recreation center.

Covered picnic tables are scattered in the shade of tall conifers. The University Hills shopping center, located 0.4 mile north of the park on Colorado Boulevard, has a coffee shop and a bagel emporium that offer outdoor relaxation at metal tables in good weather.

For more information: Denver Parks and Recreation Department, (303) 698–4903.

Getting started

Take exit 204 (South Colorado Boulevard) off I–25 and go south for 1.1 miles. Turn left (east) onto East Dartmouth Avenue and continue to the Mamie Eisenhower Park entrance on your right.

Overview

Mamie Eisenhower, wife of President Dwight D. Eisenhower, was a Denver native. She and the president often vacationed in Denver in the 1950s. The Eisenhower Recreation Center is one of six in the southeast Denver area. The park stretches for 8 blocks east from South Colorado Boulevard to South Dahlia Street and abuts the High Line Canal Trail.

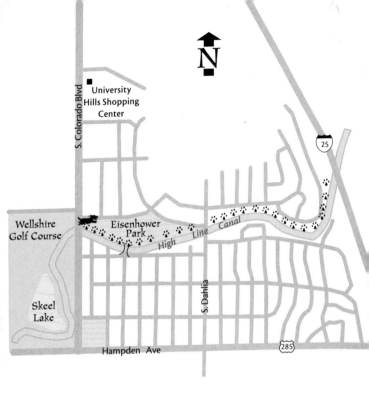

The walk

🦴 After parking your vehicle and leashing your dog, begin hiking on the south side of the parking lot that runs alongside the canal trail. There are several signs and exercise equipment stations along the perimeter of the lot that you can use to stretch your muscles before starting out.

🦴 Turn left (east) onto the canal trail and walk past the swimming pool, playground, soccer, and softball fields. The canal path is paved within Denver city limits; it's used heavily by bicyclists and occasionally by in-line skaters. Remember to keep to the right and permit bicyclists to pass on your left.

A narrow dirt footpath runs alongside the paved path along the canal bank for most of this walk, and it offers an alternative for walking during dry weather. The banks of the canal are grassy and slope gently to the water, presenting numerous places where your pet can enjoy a refreshing wallow.

🦴 At 0.2 mile a metal bridge leads to Bellaire Street. Cross South Dahlia Street and continue to South Forest Street, where another bridge connects with an urban bike route. At 0.9 mile the traffic noise from I–25 begins to intrude on the pastoral setting of tall cottonwoods, dappled shade, and the aromatic scent of wild grapevines. Farther on, the canal and the trail go under I–25, but a surface crossing on the other side of the interstate at South Holly Street and East Yale Avenue can pose problems.

🦴 Turn around at mile marker 38, which will be on the mountain side of the canal trail and denotes the distance from Waterton Canyon. Or you can pause at a nearby picnic table. Return the way you came.

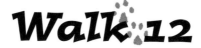

Walk 12

Bible Park

General location: Southeast Denver.

Special attractions: This is the largest park along the High Line Canal in Denver.

Open: 6 A.M. to 11 P.M.

Total distance: 1 to 3 miles round trip, depending on your starting point.

Estimated time: 30 minutes to 1½ hours.

Services: Water fountains, rest rooms, and picnic areas.

Restrictions: Your dog must be leashed.

For more information: Denver Parks and Recreation Department, (303) 698–4903.

Getting started

From I–25, take exit 202 (East Yale Avenue). Drive east on East Yale Avenue past its intersection with Monaco Parkway, a distance of about 1 mile. Bible Park is on the right (south) side of East Yale Avenue. Park in the designated area along Yale or drive another 0.1 mile to the park entrance and leave your car in the lot in the center of the horseshoe-shaped park.

Overview

Bible Park is the largest Denver park along the High Line Canal. It has picnic tables, sports fields, basketball courts, rest rooms, water, and a small, soothing, man-made waterfall just east of the parking lot where your pet can wallow in the shallows of Goldsmith Gulch Creek.

The walk

🦴 Leash your dog and, depending on where you parked, traverse a gentle upgrade to the canal trail or use the sidewalk to access

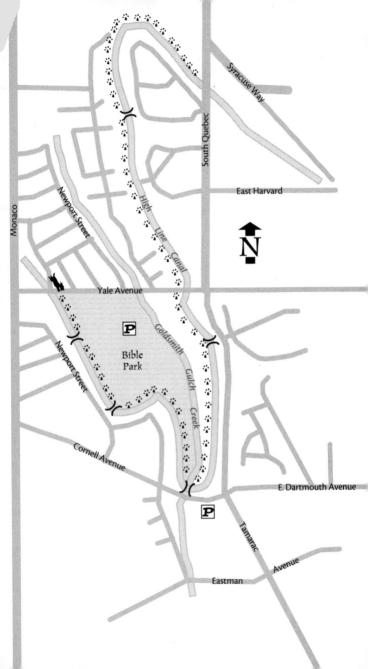

Syracuse Way

South Quebec

East Harvard

Monaco

Newport Street

N

Yale Avenue

P

Goldsmith

Bible
Park

Newport Street

Gulch

Creek

Cornell Avenue

E. Dartmouth Avenue

P

Tamarac

Avenue

Eastman

High Line Canal

the canal. Two trails loop around the park—a hard-packed dirt trail next to the canal and a paved trail at a slightly lower grade. Walkers and joggers use the dirt trail, while bicyclists and in-line skaters favor the paved path.

Having crossed Monaco Parkway and East Yale Avenue on its twisting course away from I-25 (see Walk 11), the canal makes a wide sweeping curve here as it follows the high ground of what once was the beginning of the prairie.

Four bridges link the park with local streets, and a boardwalk leads south of East Dartmouth Avenue to the Tamarac Square shopping center. The boardwalk passes through Hutchinson Park's wetlands and wildlife area. The distance around the sweeping horseshoe loop is 1 mile.

🦴 If you parked in the lot in the middle of the park, you may want to extend your hike by crossing busy East Yale Avenue (there's no pedestrian signal) to see the impressive stand of cottonwoods on the canal trail, a few hundred feet north of East Yale Avenue. These are the trees that originally sprang up along the canal trail when it was built in the 1880s. One cottonwood is at least 50 feet tall and has a trunk diameter of about 5 feet.

🦴 Ahead is a pedestrian bridge to South Olive Street. South Quebec Street is another 0.5 mile ahead. The unique character of the High Line Canal is evident in this area. Throughout its flow from the mountains, the canal remains above downtown Denver. Glimpses through the thick vegetation show the spreading city to the northwest. Return the way you came.

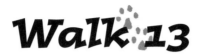

Walk 13

Potomac Street, Aurora Greenhouse, and Flower Garden

General location: Aurora.

Special attractions:
Spectacular gardens by the City of Aurora Greenhouse.

Open: 5 A.M. to 10 P.M.

Total distance: 2.4 miles round trip.

Estimated time: 45 minutes to 1¼ hours.

Services: Rest rooms, water, and picnic tables are found at nearby Del Mar Park, north of the intersection of the canal trail and Peoria Street.

Restrictions: Your dog must be on a leash. Clean up after your pet.

For more information: Aurora Parks and Open Space Department, (303) 739–7160.

Getting started

From I–225, take exit 9 (Sixth Avenue) west and continue 0.1 mile to the traffic light at Potomac Street. Turn left (south) and continue for 0.4 mile to the intersection with East Second Avenue. There is plenty of street parking.

The canal trail is just south of the spectacular block-long, flower plantings along Potomac Street by the City of Aurora Greenhouse, whose buildings abut the canal trail.

Overview

The Aurora portion of the High Line Canal became a recreational trail in 1970. Prior to that date, development near the canal toppled many old cottonwoods, so there is limited shade along the trail. This stretch of the canal runs along the Aurora Hills Golf Course, an elementary school, a middle school, and Highline Park, which has several ball fields. But the real draw is the annual planting of

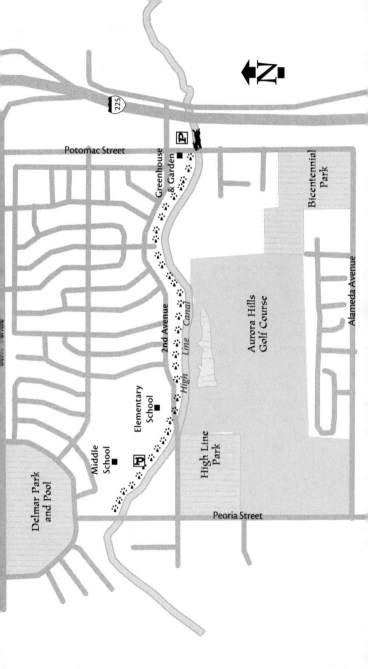

N

225

Potomac Street

Greenhouse & Garden

2nd Avenue

High Line Canal

Aurora Hills Golf Course

Bicentennial Park

Alameda Avenue

Elementary School

Middle School

Delmar Park and Pool

High Line Park

Peoria Street

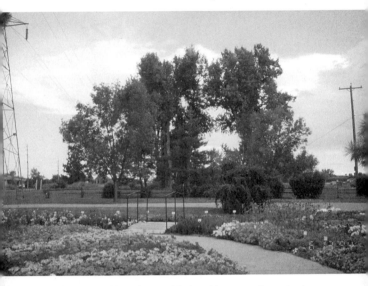

A captivating garden of annual flowers blooms against a background of tall cottonwoods on the High Line Canal in Aurora.

flowers on Potomac Street and the canal trail by the municipal greenhouse.

For this reason, this hike is best when flowers are in bloom, June to mid-September. There are two gardens. One features a hundred or so varieties of daylilies, each named with a large sign. The adjoining garden is a series of inspired plantings of annuals, from petunias to zinnias to fountain grass, in every color except black. Notice the small garden bridge that crosses an imaginary creek in the middle of the undulating beds of flowers. A large weatherproof sign at the intersection of Potomac Street and the canal depicts the canal's route through Aurora.

Walk 13 / Potomac Street, Aurora Greenhouse, and Flower Garden

The walk

🦴 After leashing your pet and admiring the flowers, pick up the canal trail and head west away of the noise of the nearby interstate. In 0.3 mile a broad grassy meadow, which is mowed regularly and tantalizingly suited for a game of Frisbee, opens on your right. The paved canal trail curves northwest around the meadow, while the narrow dirt trail used by hikers stays close to the canal bank. The meadow extends for 0.2 mile to where the paved trail swings back to the canal.

🦴 The trail runs parallel to East Second Avenue in the next 2-block-long stretch. Several locations along the open banks of the canal permit your pet easy access to water.

🦴 Continue on the trail to Peoria Street, then return the way you came.

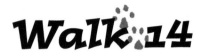

DeLaney Farm

General location: Aurora.

Special attractions: A huge
urban open space created
by a preserved homesteader's
farm; the High Line Canal;
the greenbelt; and an adjacent public golf course. Part
of the land has been returned
to the original prairie.

Open: 5 A.M. to 10 P.M.

Total distance: Several short
walks are possible in this
area, since trails crisscross the
park. Described here is a
1.3-mile loop circumnavigat-
ing the park from east to
west along the canal.

Estimated time: 45 minutes to
1¼ hours.

Services: A portable toilet and
a water spigot are available
during the growing season
near the large flower and vegetable garden (tended by volunteers) in the east portion
of the open space.

Restrictions: Your dog must be
on a leash. Clean up after
your pet.

For more information: Aurora
Parks and Open Space
Department, (303) 739–7160.

Getting started

From I–225 take exit 7 (East Mississippi Avenue) east for 0.9 mile to
its intersection with Chambers Road. Turn north (left) and continue
for 1 mile to the entrance to the DeLaney Farm on your right, just
short of the intersection with East Sixth Avenue. There is a small
paved parking lot near one of the barns.

Overview

This is a huge urban open space that offers a variety of experiences,
from a glimpse of life on the prairie a hundred years ago to scenic
views of the Front Range and a visit to a prairie dog town. Your

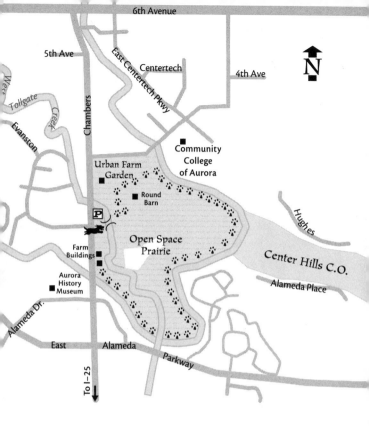

options include walking on a narrow path adjacent to a restored prairie meadow and strolling next to a golf course on a modern, paved path.

The most historically notable building is the large, round white barn in the middle of the former farm. Constructed around 1902, it served as a grain storage silo, then in 1912 was converted into a two-story cow barn. The barn is considered the only surviving perfectly round barn in Colorado. Its exceptional construction and engineering are believed to have been the work of an itinerant carpenter.

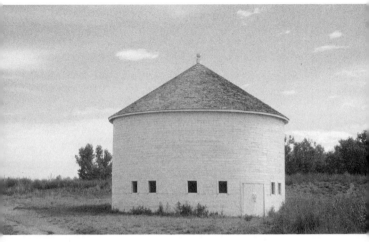

This round barn is part of the DeLaney Farm homestead.

The John DeLaney family lived in the frame house near the entrance to the parking lot from Chambers Road.

The small house to the right (south) at the edge of the property along Chambers Road is the Gully house, named for an Irish family that immigrated to Colorado in 1862. One of their eight children was Bridget, who married John DeLaney.

The walk

🦴 After leashing your dog, examine the two houses and the half-dozen outbuildings, some of which have been transported here from other locations in Aurora that were developed. As you face the round barn in the meadow, you'll see several paths through the property as well as the High Line Canal in the distance to your right.

🦴 To make a 1.3-mile loop around the open space by using

the distant High Line Canal Trail for part of your walk, cross West Tollgate Creek on the bridge before you. Continue on the dirt path past the round barn and on to the urban farm community beyond it. (This is where you'll find a portable toilet and a spigot for water during the growing season.)

🦴 Skirt the garden to the east and then continue on the narrow path in a northeast direction to a stand of trees. The path veers to the right, goes down into a gulch created by East Tollgate Creek, and crosses the creek on a wooden bridge that connects with the High Line Canal Trail. Turn right (west) on the paved canal trail.

You'll pass the buildings of Aurora Community College, then the Centre Hill Golf Course, before emerging onto a broad sweep of the canal trail around a large meadow. The meadow, once part of the DeLaney farm, has been restored to a prairie. Keep close watch on your dog here, because there's a small colony of prairie dogs in the area. Ahead of you, the Front Range rises into the blue Colorado sky.

🦴 Continue to the point where the canal trail crosses West Tollgate Creek on a pedestrian bridge, then follow the trail as it approaches Chambers Road. The last 50 yards of the walk are on a broad sidewalk along the east side of Chambers Road as you again approach the buildings on the DeLaney farm from the south.

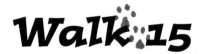

Walk 15

Discovery Pavilion

General location: Off South Wadsworth Boulevard in Jefferson County at the mouth of Waterton Canyon.

Special attractions: Scenic views and excellent interpretive signs.

Total distance: 2.5 miles round trip.

Estimated time: 1 to 1½ hours.

Services: Drinking water and rest rooms at Discovery Pavilion.

Restrictions: Your dog must be on a leash.

For more information: Chatfield State Park, (303) 791–7275.

Getting started

From C–470 south of Denver, take the South Wadsworth Boulevard exit. Go south on Wadsworth Boulevard (C–121) for 4.5 miles to the marked turnoff for Waterton Canyon. Turn left (east) onto Waterton Road, then take the first left, which leads into the Discovery Pavilion parking lot. The trail begins at the northwest corner of the parking lot.

Overview

The Discovery Pavilion was dedicated in August 1997 and is said to be the only spot in the country where three major recreational trails converge: the Colorado Trail, the High Line Canal Trail, and the Platte River Greenway Trail. The Colorado Trail begins across Waterton Road and is served by a second parking lot immediately south of the Discovery Pavilion. No pets are allowed in Waterton Canyon due to efforts to protect a herd of bighorn sheep. The Colorado Trail is at Waterton Road. The High Line Canal is not accessible to the public in the canyon. The Discovery Pavilion marks

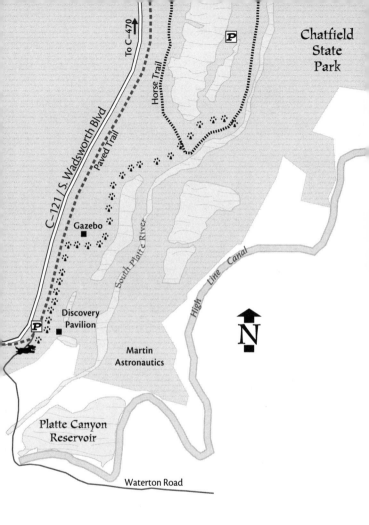

the start of the Platte River Greenway Trail, although there are no mile markers or directional signs for the greenway trail. The trail runs along South Wadsworth Boulevard and approximately 0.5 mile west of the river itself. Interpretive signs at the rotunda outside the pavilion describe the three trails.

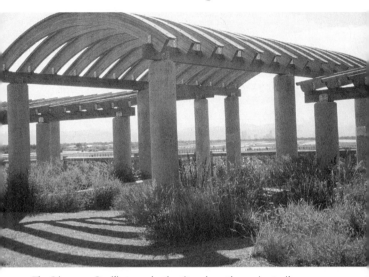

The Discovery Pavilion marks the site where the major trails come together.

The walk

🦴 After putting your dog on a leash, begin at the northwest corner of the parking lot and follow the broad, paved trail for 0.6 mile. The trail parallels South Wadsworth Boulevard and can be noisy in this stretch. Leave the noise behind by turning right onto a wide footpath to the clearly visible gazebo overlooking a series of ponds and marshes.

The ponds were created as water reuse ponds by Lockheed Martin, the aeronautics plant upstream of the river. Today the wetlands cover twelve acres and support muskrats, paddle ducks, avocets, and herons. This area is administered by the park.

🦴 From the gazebo, continue on a footpath along the marshy, low bank of the pond, which offers several places where your pet can wallow at the sandy bank. The footpath ends at a jeep road. A sign marks the original boundary of Chatfield State Park, before it was extended into Lockheed Martin land.

🦴 Continue right (east) on the jeep road, past a turnoff for a parking lot on your left, until you reach the South Platte River amid lush vegetation of willows and cottonwoods. A narrow angler's trail runs southward along the bank of the river, and a horse trail runs north. If the ground is wet and puddled, portions of the path may be under water and impassable in either direction. Watch your footing.

The area adjoining the river consists of several open meadows and low brush belts with active bird life. Bald eagles, great blue herons, Canada geese, as well as foxes and deer have been spotted in these areas.

🦴 Turn around and return the way you came. If you want to make a loop by following the riverbank south, see Walk 16.

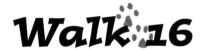

Walk 16

Discovery Pavilion, River Route

General location: Discovery Pavilion is located at the mouth of Waterton Canyon, off South Wadsworth Boulevard in Jefferson County.

Special attractions: Scenic views and excellent interpretive signs.

Total distance: 2 miles round trip.

Estimated time: 40 minutes to 1 hour.

Services: Drinking water and rest rooms at Discovery Pavilion.

Restrictions: Your dog must be on a leash.

For more information: Chatfield State Park, (303) 791–7275.

Getting started

From C–470 south of Denver, take the South Wadsworth Boulevard exit. Go south on South Wadsworth Boulevard (C–121) for 4.5 miles to the marked turnoff for Waterton Canyon. Turn left (east) onto Waterton Road, then take the first left, which leads into the Discovery Pavilion parking lot.

Overview

The Discovery Pavilion and the ponds and wetlands immediately to the north are the result of a partnership led by the Lockheed Martin Astronautics Foundation, public agencies, and private citizens, including 300 volunteers who planted hundreds of trees and shrubs in the area around the pavilion in the spring of 1996.

Standing on the banks of one of the ponds and surveying the dozen acres of adjacent marshland with its active bird life, it's hard to imagine that westward and behind a hill, vehicles are being assembled that boost spacecraft to other planets. Lockheed Martin

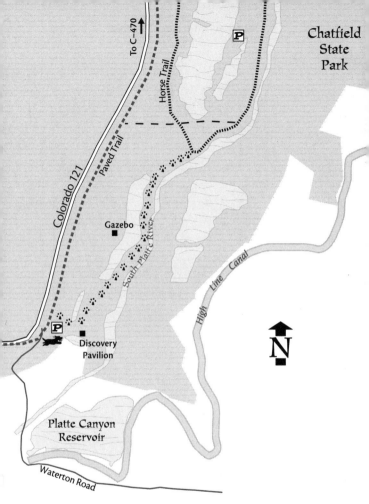

has built rockets for the Viking, Voyager, Magellan, Galileo, and Pathfinder space probes. The wetland area is administered by Chatfield State Park.

The walk

🦴 After leashing your dog, begin at the parking lot's northeast corner (a sign says FISHING, with an arrow pointing to the right).

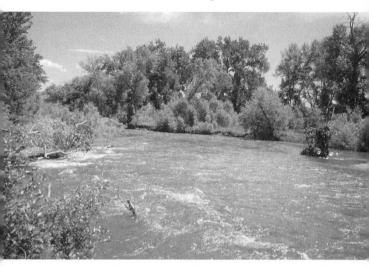

The South Platte River flows fast and free as it approaches Chatfield Dam.

Follow a narrow footpath with the pond on your left and head east toward a stand of tall cottonwoods. This is the widest of several footpaths that lead from the parking lot to the banks of the South Platte River; they're used by anglers fishing for bass, trout, and pike along the river's low banks.

As the footpath nears the river, the vegetation becomes thick and lush. At places, willows droop over the footpath. The footpath ends at the sandy, low bank of the river where your pet will have access to the water.

🦴 Follow the path north along the riverbank for up to 1.5 miles, through thick vegetation and dense stands of willow. After rainfall or during wet seasons, sections of the path may be under water. This footpath is not heavily used; you'll be pretty much alone. Turn around and return the way you came.

Optional loop

To create a loop, follow the riverbank for 1.5 miles. Look for a horse trail, then a jeep road to your left leading away from the river. Continue on the jeep road for 0.3 mile, past a parking lot on your right. Proceed on the jeep road as it passes a pond on the left. Beyond the pond, look for a footpath along the pond's west bank and follow it south to the gazebo overlook described in Walk 15. From the gazebo, pick up the paved trail and continue south on the greenway trail to the parking lot at Discovery Pavilion.

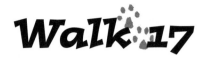

Walk 17

Chatfield State Park

General location: South end of Chatfield State Park, off South Wadsworth Boulevard (C–121), Jefferson County.

Special attractions: Picnic areas, scenic views, horse stables, and a marina.

Open: The park is open year-round, but facilities such as the marina and horse stables operate April through October, 9 A.M. to 5 P.M.

Total distance: 3 miles round trip.

Estimated time: 1 to 1½ hours.

Services: Rest rooms (closed during the winter months) at the parking lot.

Restrictions: You'll need a daily pass or an annual permit to enter the park by car. Dogs must be on a leash.

For more information: Chatfield State Park, (303) 791–7275

Getting started

From C–470 south of Denver, take the South Wadsworth Boulevard exit. Go south on South Wadsworth Boulevard (C–121) to the marked turnoff for Chatfield State Park. Turn left and drive to the park entrance. After leaving the entrance booth, proceed to a stop sign. Turn right (south) and continue for 2 miles. Cross the bridge over the South Platte River and park in the parking lot on your right, just past the bridge.

Overview

The South Platte River hasn't been dammed yet, and it's a brisk, fast flowing river as it heads downstream to the Chatfield Reservoir and Dam. The low rumble of the current is audible as the trail leads from the parking lot to a narrow pathway that follows the easterly bank of the river. Stands of towering cottonwoods block out the sky,

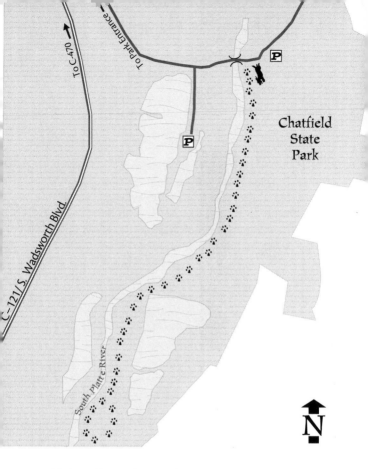

while box elders and willows form dense underbrush. Occasionally the river spills out into an oxbow with shallow banks and quiet pools of water, which your pet will welcome. Because the path is narrow, leads through thick underbrush, and has two steep sections, it's a moderately difficult walk.

The walk

🦴 After putting your dog on a leash, begin by scrambling down the slope to an old rutted jeep road on the other side of the handicapped parking spaces. A concrete bench and a wide concrete walk that butt up to the west side of the jeep road are part of a fishing access trail for the handicapped.

🦴 Turn left (south) onto the jeep road and look for a wide footpath to your right that runs to the riverbank and continues south. The riverbank first rises in elevation, then dips down into marshland.

🦴 Continue for 1 mile to the larger of two ponds, where you may encounter anglers. Follow the trail between the ponds and the river for another 0.5 mile to a large meadow crisscrossed by several footpaths. The footpath ends just beyond the meadow in a marshy area. Turn around and return the way you came.

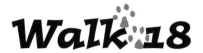

South Platte Park

General location: Littleton.
Special attractions:
Wide-open spaces, a nature
preserve, a wildflower garden,
and a nature center.
Open: Sunrise to sunset.
Total distance: 4.6 miles round
trip, although a shuttle is pos-
sible.
Estimated time: 2 to 3 hours.
Services: Rest rooms, benches,
and water fountains.

Restrictions: Your dog must be
on a leash.
For more information: South
Suburban Park and
Recreation District, (303)
789–5131; Carson Nature
Center, (303) 730–1022. (The
center is open Tuesday
through Friday noon to 4:30
P.M., and Saturday and Sunday
9:30 A.M. to 4:30 P.M.)

Getting started

There are two access points for this walk. You can start at the South
Suburban Tennis and Golf Club on South Federal Boulevard, just
west of Santa Fe Drive at the intersection of West Bowles Avenue
and South Federal Boulevard, or you can set off from the Carson
Nature Center, just north of West Mineral Avenue.

If you'd like to do this picturesque segment of the Platte River
Greenway as a shuttle, leave one car at the nature center. To reach
the center, take Santa Fe Drive south to West Mineral Avenue, then
turn right (west) and go past the RTD parking lot. Turn right (north)
onto Platte River Parkway and follow signs to the nature center and
the adjoining parking lot.

To access the parking at South Federal Boulevard, return to
Santa Fe and drive north for 2.3 miles to its intersection with West
Bowles Avenue. Turn left (west) and continue for 0.3 mile to the
intersection with South Federal Boulevard. Turn right (north) and

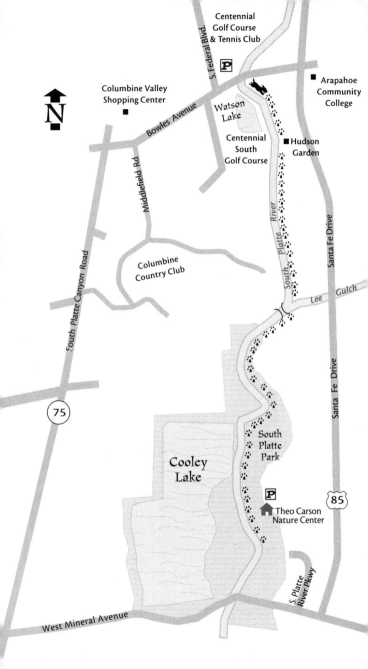

N

Centennial Golf Course & Tennis Club

S. Federal Blvd

Columbine Valley Shopping Center

Bowles Avenue

Watson Lake

Centennial South Golf Course

Arapahoe Community College

Hudson Garden

South Platte River

Middlefield Rd

Columbine Country Club

Lee Gulch

Santa Fe Drive

South Platte Canyon Road

75

South Platte Park

Cooley Lake

Santa Fe Drive

85

Theo Carson Nature Center

S. Platte River Pkwy

West Mineral Avenue

park in the lot on your right that's used by the South Suburban Tennis and Golf Club

Overview

The centerpiece of this hike is South Platte Park, which has been thirty years in the making, ever since the U.S. Army Corps of Engineers proposed the Chatfield Dam and Reservoir project after a devastating flood in 1965. The corps also proposed to channelize the river through the city of Littleton. Following objections by local residents, the city's efforts to preserve the floodplain resulted in the passage of the 1974 Water Resources Development Act. This legislation set a national precedent by requiring the Corps of Engineers to participate in development of floodplain parks as an alternative to channelization. South Platte Park was created as a result of this legislation. In the decades that followed, the dam was built and the city of Littleton began acquiring land along the river and eliminating gravel mining. The park you see today was assembled one parcel at a time and now encompasses 650 acres.

The floodplain, extensively gravel mined since the 1950s, was painstakingly reclaimed. Today the largest gravel pit is a lake, and the land and water quality has been restored so that the habitat supports more than 225 species of birds and 23 species of fish.

The city of Littleton owns the land, while the South Suburban Park and Recreation District administers the park.

The walk

The walk begins at the South Suburban Tennis and Golf Club because the parking lot at Riverfront Center, the former store arcade on the south side of West Bowles Avenue, is no longer available. Riverfront Center has been sold to Echo Star, a satellite dish company, and the once public parking lots are now private.

After leashing your dog, head to the right of the covered tennis pavilion on a concrete sidewalk used by golfers and tennis players. The sidewalk intersects with the greenway trail. Turn right (south) onto the trail and proceed through an underpass under West Bowles Avenue to access the trail south of West Bowles Avenue.

In this area the greenway is designated the Arapahoe Greenway, which was dedicated in 1988. Several memorials along the way mention people and organizations that helped make this portion of the greenbelt along the Platte possible.

🦴 At 0.2 mile pass Hudson Gardens, an arboretum with sixteen distinct gardens, on your left.

A refreshment pavilion with outdoor tables and chairs fronts on the river. This is a pleasant place to stop for a soda or an ice cream on a hot summer day. The gently sloping bank offers several places where your pet can go down to the water's edge for a wallow.

🦴 At 1 mile into the walk, the path intersects with the Lee Gulch Trail, which connects the Platte to the High Line Canal (see Walk 3). Just past the intersection is the start of South Platte Park; the boundary is marked with a sign, a bench, and a commemorative plaque. Beyond the bench, a path leads to the river's edge, where there's a tiny sand beach. The river bottom is sandy and flat here.

Once you're inside the South Platte Park area, note the nature preserve along the river. The Cooley Gravel Company ended mining in 1989, and the land was reclaimed into a lake and adjoining wildlife preserve. The greenway trail swings east and away from the river at this point. To protect the wildlife habitat around Cooley Lake, the area is closed except for ranger-led hikes. An eighteen-acre buffer zone, added in 1997 between the river and Santa Fe Drive, keeps the rumble of the highway and the development in Arapahoe County at bay.

🦴 You'll reach the Carson Nature Center 2.3 miles from where you started. This center has exhibits on local history and environment. The building is a hand-built log home moved to its present site in 1986. Rest rooms, a drinking fountain, an observation deck, bird feeders, and a wildflower garden make the center a pleasant rest area. South Platte Park continues for another 1.5 miles to C–470 and the Centennial Trail.

Return the way you came, or pick up your car if you've opted for a shuttle walk. If you return to Bowles Avenue, the Pitchers Sports Bar next to the Riverfront Center caters to trail users and has an outdoor patio in good weather.

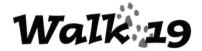

Walk 19

Ruby Hill Park Area

General location: West Denver.

Special attractions: A pond, a historic area, and 360-degree view.

Open: 5 A.M. to 11 P.M.

Total distance: 1.8 miles round trip, 2.3 miles if you climb Ruby Hill.

Estimated time: 1 to 2 hours.

Services: Portable toilet near the pond; rest rooms and water at Pasquinel's Landing and Ruby Hill Parks.

Restrictions: Your dog must be on a leash. Pick up after your pet. Keep to the right to enable bicyclists and in-line skaters to pass.

For more information: Denver Department of Parks and Recreation, (303) 698–4903.

Getting started

From Santa Fe Drive, take the Evans Avenue exit heading west. Go 2 blocks on West Evans Avenue to the first traffic light. This is South Huron Street. Turn right (north) and continue to West Asbury Drive, then turn into a parking lot by the playground in Pasquinel's Landing Park.

Overview

This segment of the Platte River Greenway is worth a visit, especially if you're a fan of James Michener. The park is named for one of the most engaging characters in Michener's *Centennial*, the story of the land that became Colorado. Pasquinel is a French trapper who fearlessly goes into Colorado and Wyoming to hunt beaver, then transports his bounty by harnessing himself to the bundled pelts and dragging them across half a continent. Just north of the park is the Overland Golf Course, which creates a buffer between the

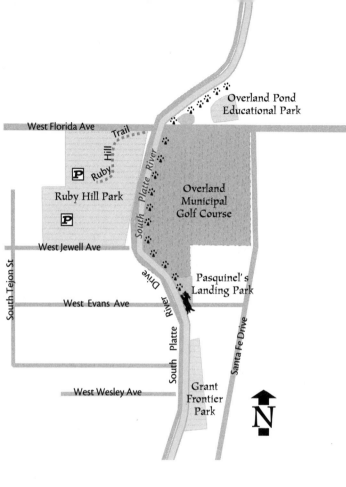

West Florida Ave

Overland Pond
Educational Park

Ruby Hill Trail

P

Ruby Hill Park

P

South Platte River

Overland
Municipal
Golf Course

West Jewell Ave

South Tejon St

South Platte River Drive

Pasquinel's
Landing Park

West Evans Ave

South Platte River

Santa Fe Drive

West Wesley Ave

Grant
Frontier
Park

N

greenway and busy Santa Fe Drive. The side trip to Ruby Hill offers
a 360-degree view of the metro area.

The walk ends at Overland Pond, which was once a quarry
owned by the city of Denver. There are several places where your
pet has access to the water and can frolic in the sandy shallows
near the bank.

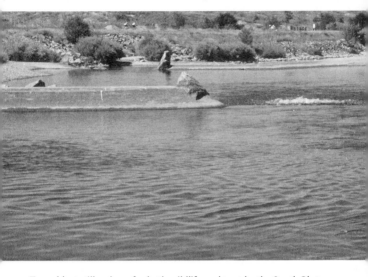

Tamed but still a draw for both wildlife and people, the South Platte River makes it's way through Denver.

The walk

🦴 The Platte River Greenway trail runs along the west side of Pasquinel's Landing Park. After putting your dog on a leash, turn right (north) on the trail. Almost immediately the Overland Golf Course, separated from the trail by a fence, begins on your right.

The Platte's banks slope gently to the water, and there are patches of grass that make the river accessible. This is a calm portion of the river without strong currents or rapids.

This is one of the most historic areas of Denver. The Arapahoe and the Ute camped at the foot of Ruby Hill, which, because of its height, was a good lookout over the prairie. After the arrival of settlers, the land was a potato farm, then in 1883 became a park to which the Denver Circle Railway Company ran an excursion train. Subsequently a racecourse was built in the vicinity, then an auto racecourse. During World War I the park was a military camp. The golf course was built in the 1930s and is a municipal facility.

〰️At 0.7 mile you'll reach the greenway trail's intersection with West Florida Avenue. Here you'll find a junction with the Sanderson Gulch Trail, which leads to Ruby Hill Park. Ruby Hill is one of the highest points in Denver, rising 100 feet above the river. Early prospectors found small red garnets along the river that they thought were rubies.

If you plan to ascend Ruby Hill, turn left (west) on West Florida Avenue and continue across the bridge to South Platte River Drive, which has a pedestrian crossing signal. Walk 0.2 mile up the hill to a sign for Ruby Hill Park. Make a sharp left on the cement path that leads to the top of the hill. You can also drive up to the top by using a road that begins at West Florida Avenue, just past the cement path. The road has a gate that's closed at night and during bad weather.

If you don't plan to make the side trip to Ruby Hill, there's no pedestrian crossing sign at West Florida Avenue and the greenway. There is, however, an underpass that you can use to cross the avenue. The underpass path veers to the left from the main path as you approach the avenue.

〰️From West Florida Avenue, you can continue north for another 0.2 mile by crossing the street to Overland Pond Educational Park, where there are several interpretive signs.

Farther north, the greenway trail runs past the Gates Rubber Company plant and a number of warehouses. When Santa Fe Drive ends at I–25, the river and the trail are sandwiched between the interstate and South Platte River Drive until the trail reaches the Public Service generating plant, just south of Mile High Stadium. North of the stadium the trail runs on both sides of the river, then comes together at Confluence Park (see Walk 20).

〰️Turn around and return the way you came.

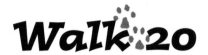

Walk 20

Confluence Park to City of Cuernavaca Park

General location: Denver's lower downtown.

Special attractions: Views of the Denver skyline, Union Station, and Coors Field.

Open: 5 A.M. to 11 P.M.

Total distance: 2.3 miles round trip.

Estimated time: 1½ to 2 hours.

Services: None.

Restrictions: Your dog must be on a leash. Pick up after your pet. Keep to the right to enable bicyclists and in-line skaters to pass. There's a two-hour parking limit at the Fishback Landing parking lot.

For more information: Denver Department of Parks and Recreation, (303) 698–4903.

Getting started

Take exit 211 off I–25. At the top of the ramp, turn right and follow Water Street past the Ocean Journey Aquarium to a parking lot along the Platte River that serves Fishback Landing Park. A sign tells you that parking is restricted to two hours.

From downtown Denver, take Fifteenth Street west. Turn left onto Platte Street, go under the Speer Boulevard viaduct, and park in the Fishback Landing lot on your left.

Overview

This loop walk starts just short of Confluence Park, continues north along the South Platte River Greenway, and returns on a concrete path completed in 2000 on the opposite side (east bank) of the river, where old railroad yards are being reclaimed for housing, offices, and two parks. Although it's close to I–25—with several overpasses above the greenway path that connect the downtown

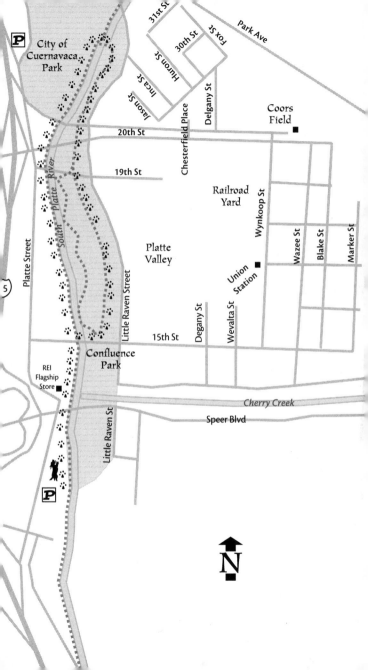

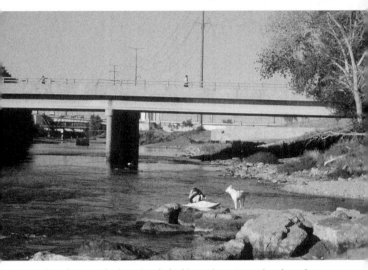

A kayaker, watched anxiously by his canine companion, launches his kayak at the confluence of the South Platte River and Cherry Creek.

to the interstate—the walk is peaceful, because rapids along the river drown out highway noise. In addition, the walk offers unusual vistas of the downtown area, of Union Station, and of the baseball diamond in Coors Field. Despite construction of the parks on the east bank of the river, the area remains little known and is not heavily frequented.

The walk

🦴 After parking at the Fishback Landing lot and putting your dog on a leash, turn left (north) and follow the concrete path into Confluence Park. If you haven't been here before, cross over on a pedestrian bridge to the other bank and notice the sign on the grassy knoll. The side facing west says PLATTE RIVER GREENWAY, while the back of the sign says CHERRY CREEK GREENWAY.

This is the confluence of two of Colorado's most famous bodies of water, Cherry Creek and the South Platte River. Gold was discovered here in 1858, prompting the gold rush in Colorado. Confluence Park is also a monument to changes in the way we think about the use of the river and creek. For most of the twentieth century, both streams served as sewage and garbage dumps. Industries along the banks further polluted and degraded both waterways.

Earth Day 1970 began the slow revitalization of these streams. Confluence Park, with ramps to the water, an amphitheater, and several overlooks high above the confluence, was dedicated as a symbol that Denver and its neighbors were committed to saving the waterways.

🐾 After looking down at the turbulence caused by the mingling of two waterways, retrace your steps over the pedestrian crosswalk, turn right (north), and begin your walk. Stop and read the plaque at Shoemaker Plaza, which honors Joe Shoemaker, the chairman of the Greenway Foundation, who was a catalyst for the restoration of the South Platte.

The huge redbrick building on your left was built in 1901 by the Denver Tramway Power Company and served as a trolley yard and, more recently, as the Forney Railroad Museum. The museum moved to Golden, and was replaced by the Colorado flagship store for REI, a sporting goods and outdoor recreation chain.

🐾 After passing the Fifteenth Street viaduct, the trail descends to the banks of the Platte. There are several places where your dog can have a romp.

🐾 The next overpass is the Nineteenth Street viaduct. Next to it is a pedestrian bridge. If you want to cut your walk short, cross here to the other side. Pass a second pedestrian bridge just past the Twentieth Street viaduct and the ramp from I–25 to Coors Field. You can also cross to the other side here if you want to shorten your outing.

🐾 Otherwise continue through the City of Cuernavaca Park

toward the Park Avenue viaduct in the distance. Before this overpass, the trail ends in a barricade. Beyond the barricade, a dirt path continues for a few hundred feet. This is another good place to let your dog frolic in the water: The bank is flat, and there are no bicyclists.

🦴 Return to the barricade and follow a concrete ramp that leads to the third, and last, pedestrian bridge. Cross the river to the east side of the City of Cuernavaca Park. Follow the concrete path through the park. Notice the two sculptures on a grassy lawn that sweeps down to the water. Both look like miniature Stonehenges—hewn rock columns arranged in semicircles.

🦴 Follow the concrete past the distant facade of Union Station. After passing the Twentieth Street overpass, you'll be in Commons Park. Several places slope down gently to the water. There is also a sand-and-pebble beachlike area just behind a pavilion built in 2000. There are numerous benches in this area as well as a curved granite staircase that leads from the pavilion to a concrete path, which in turn takes you to the riverbank. Follow either the lower or the upper concrete path through the park, and then use the concrete ramps to rise to the Fifteenth Street viaduct. The ramps lead to the sidewalk on the viaduct.

🦴 After crossing the Platte River, turn right and use the ramp to descend to the concrete path. Complete the loop the way you came.

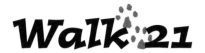

Walk 21

East Eighty-Eighth Avenue to McKay Road

General location: Thornton.

Special attractions: Distant views of Denver's skyline, open stretches of the South Platte River, and a working farm alongside the trail.

Open: Sunrise to sunset.

Total distance: 4.6 miles round trip.

Estimated time: 2½ to 3 hours.

Services: Rest rooms, water, and picnic tables.

Restrictions: Your dog must be on a leash. Keep to the right, and let bicyclists and in-line skaters pass you safely on your left.

For more information: Adams County Park and Recreation Department, (303) 637–8000; Thornton Parks and Recreation Department, (303) 538–7300.

Getting started

From I–25 north of Denver, take I–76 east, getting off at the East Eighty-eighth Avenue exit. Go west on Eighty-eighth Avenue through two traffic lights to Colorado Boulevard. Turn left and park in the lot at Trailhead Park on your left. The park is adjacent to the city of Thornton's municipal service center and water treatment plant.

Overview

From Cuernavaca Park west of Union Station in LoDo and north to where the Platte receives the waters of Clear Creek, the river and the greenway trail pass through a heavily industrialized area that includes stockyards, a municipal sewage treatment plant, a Public Service plant, and a refinery.

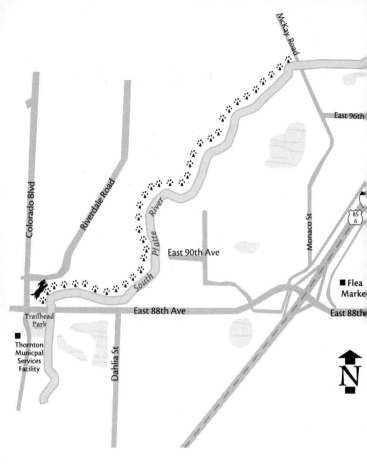

The junction of the South Platte and Clear Creek is near I–76 and 0.5 mile from I–270, so this is a rather noisy area. On July 5, 1820, Maj. Stephen Long's expedition camped here. This is also the spot where, in 1832, Fort Convenience—the first trading post north of the Arkansas River—was built on the east bank of the Platte opposite the mouth of Clear Creek.

Farther downstream, the heavy concentration of industrial activity eases as the river curves northeast and begins its course across the prairie. The land becomes flat and open. The walker gets a

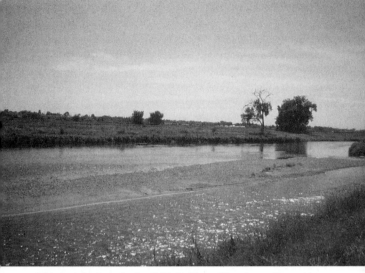

This stretch along the South Platte River offers dog walkers wide open vistas of river and prairie.

glimpse of the broad, free-flowing river meandering across the shortgrass prairie. The banks are low and gentle in this area, with numerous sandbars in the river that connect to an occasional sandy beach.

This area was once the agricultural center for Denver. Today there are still some small farms—one right along the trail farther downstream.

The greenway is completed up to McKay Road. Land along the river is being acquired under an ambitious plan adopted in 1997 by Adams County; eventually the greenway trail will run uninterrupted to Brighton. Construction of the greenway north of McKay Road began in 2000.

The walk

🦴 After leashing your dog, cross the park to the river and turn left (northeast) on the concrete trail.

The Platte is shallow and broad here, and has been extensively mined for gravel. One of the operators in this area is the Cooley Gravel Company, which had a large gravel operation on the Platte at what is now South Platte Park in Littleton (See Walk 18). Abandoned gravel pits are being redeveloped as water storage lakes for Thornton, and as wildlife habitats similar to South Platte Park. However, gravel mining is still ongoing, and you can hear the rumble of conveyor belts.

🦴 Pass a small farm; a corral adjacent to the trail is inhabited by a flock of speckled goats. Beyond it is a large chicken coop.

🦴 The trail ends at McKay Road. Turn around and return the way you came.

On your way back, the skyline of Denver, rising against the purple bulk of the distant mountains, dominates the horizon to the southwest. Ducks and other waterfowl, including gulls, can be seen preening on sandbars in the shallow water. There are many places where the thick underbrush of willows recedes and the riverbank is open and low, offering your pet easy access to the water.

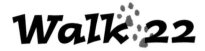

Walk 22

Adams County Regional Park

General location: Brighton.

Special attractions: This is the final stretch of greenway trail to the north.

Open: Sunrise to sunset.

Total distance: 2 miles round trip on the greenway; add 0.8 mile for a loop around the lake.

Estimated time: 1½ to 2 hours.

Services: Rest rooms and picnic tables.

Restrictions: Your dog must be on a leash.

For more information: Adams County Park and Recreation Department, (303) 637–8000.

Getting started

From I–25 north of Denver, take I–76 east for 7.2 miles to the point where it branches off in a V. Take the left arm of the V, marked U.S. 85 NORTH/EXIT 12 BRIGHTON. Take Route 85 to the second traffic light; this is East 124th Avenue. Turn left (west) and drive for about a mile. The road name changes to Henderson Road at a four-way stop sign at Brighton Road. Continue past the stop sign, cross the South Platte River, and continue a few hundred feet. A turnoff on your right leads into a parking lot overlooking a large lake.

Overview

This walk takes you into Adams County Regional Park, a multiuse facility that includes fairgrounds on the west and a campground to the north. Extending the Platte River Greenway through Adams County is a project that has gained momentum. One of the sections finished in 1998 is the 1-mile stretch in the park. This project was funded by the Colorado Lottery.

The Brighton area is still rural, with dairy and vegetable farms, as well as gravel quarries near the river. The land is flat; the mountains

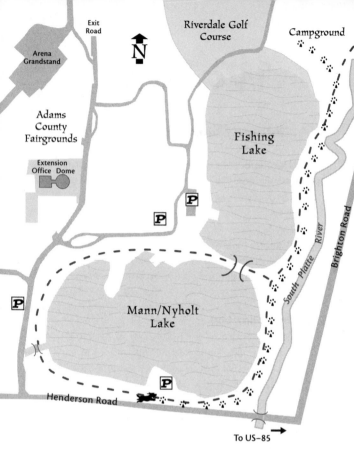

are mere shadows on the western horizon. This walk thus offers a refreshing change of pace from the dynamic activity of the metro area. Mann/Nyholt Lake and the adjacent lake—simply called Fishing Lake—are stocked with bass and popular with local anglers. It's not unusual to see bass jumping out of the water to catch flies.

The walk

After parking your car and putting your dog on a leash, pick up the dirt trail on the east side of the parking lot. This trail

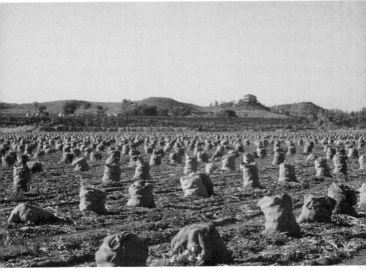

Onions, sacked and ready for shipment to market, dot a field alongside the South Platte River in Brighton.

ends in the paved greenway trail, which runs along the bank of the Platte River.

If you turn right (south) here, the trail ends after it goes under the Henderson Road overpass. It becomes a jeep road that passes an active gravel pit on the right, then a large cultivated field where onions are grown commercially. Beyond the field, the dirt road veers away from the river and heads for farm buildings.

The trail north is a more quiet and scenic walk. It skirts the lakes on the left, then the fifteenth tee of the Riverdale Golf Course, before petering out in the campground. While you walk next to Fishing Lake, the river is immediately to your right, its banks gentle and low. Beyond the lake, the trail veers away from the river. Turn around and return the way you came.

Alternate route

For a longer outing, on the way back turn right (west) onto a clearly defined concrete footpath that leads to a footbridge between the lakes. Follow the trail to the left (southwest) as it circles the shoreline of Mann/Nyholt Lake. The trail turns to dirt past a small fishing pier. There are two more footbridges to cross. Eventually, your trail narrows into a angler's path, running alongside Henderson Road for several hundred yards before reaching the parking lot.

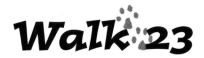

Walk 23

Confluence Park

General location: Downtown Denver.

Special attractions: A pedestrians-only trail along the Cherry Creek Greenway.

Open: 5 A.M. to 11 P.M.

Total distance: 1.8 miles round trip.

Estimated time: 45 minutes to 1 hour.

Services: None.

Restrictions: Your dog must be on a leash. Clean up after your pet.

For more information: Denver Parks and Recreation Department, (303) 698–4903.

Getting started

From I–25, take exit 210C (Colfax Avenue) to Speer Boulevard. Stay in the left lane. As soon as you cross Speer, make a quick left onto Welton Street. There is adequate street parking on Welton near the Emily Griffith Opportunity School and at a parking lot between Colfax and Welton.

Overview

Starting at Colfax Avenue and continuing for nearly a mile to Confluence Park, the Cherry Creek Greenway offers separate trails for walkers and bicyclists. The greenway trail divides just past the Colfax Avenue overpass, where bicyclists and in-line skaters are diverted across the creek on a pedestrian bridge, while the path on the east side is set aside exclusively for pedestrians. The Creekside Landing at Larimer Street is on the pedestrian path and offers you a respite on a broad series of concrete ledges that descend to the water's edge.

Larimer is arguably the most famous of Denver's streets. A plaque

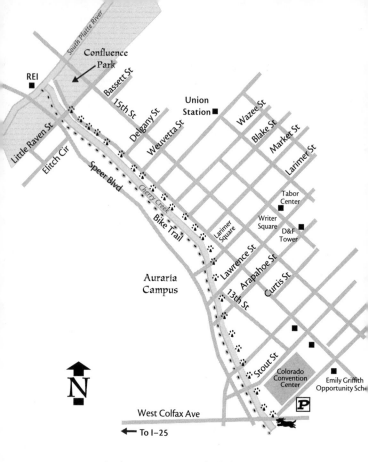

commemorates its importance. It reads: "While he diplomatically named the frontier town for territorial governor James Denver, Gen. William H. Larimer named its major street for himself. It survived fires, floods and explosive growth. The hotels, bars, stores and amusements of the granite-lined thoroughfare were a barometer of the regional boom. The bust that began with the 1893 silver crash continued into the depression and beyond. Elegant Larimer Street became skid row, home to depleted miners, busted sodbusters and worn out cowboys and Indians. As Denver moved 'uptown,' tolerant Larimer Street became a magnet for immigrants—Mexican,

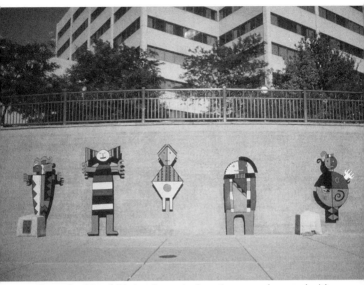

The walls of Creekside Landing at Larimer Street are decorated with Native American motifs.

Japanese, African, German, Irish, Italian and Jews. Urban renewal in the 1970s erased much of the brick and sandstone in Larimer Street's history but today the rejuvenated street again measures Denver's urban renaissance."

The walk

🐾🦴 After parking your car and putting your dog on a leash, cross the westbound lanes of Speer Boulevard at the traffic signal at Colfax Avenue. Once you're in the center median strip, turn right and descend on the ramp to the creek path. Turn right.

This is the beginning of walkers only path: Bicyclists and in-line skaters are diverted across the creek by clearly marked signs. The creekside greenway is beautifully landscaped here, with regularly mowed, lawnlike banks sweeping gently to the water where your pet can access the water easily.

The Creekside Landing at Larimer Street is worth a stop. Examine the sculptures on the granite wall. Wide, deep ledges lead down to the water. It's not unusual to see a student from Auraria Campus across the street studying at the water's edge while dangling bare toes into the water. If you have a yen for refreshments, this area has many outdoor cafes that do not object to well-behaved dogs.

🦴 Go up the stairs to street level to reach Larimer Street. Turn right and walk to Fifteenth Street. Cross at the traffic signal to the pocket park in the triangle formed by the diagonally running Speer Boulevard and downtown streets. The large bell in the park is the only remaining artifact of Denver's original city hall, which stood on this spot until it was razed in 1936.

🦴 Turn right, cross Fifteenth Street, and enter famous Larimer Square, the first block of downtown to be reclaimed back in the 1970s.

The Market Café and the Mexicali Café up the block on the left have outdoor tables. The Market is famous for its coffee drinks and for its desserts. Light lunch or dinner entrees are also available. The Mexicali Café serves Mexican fare. You'll also find a Starbucks.

🦴 If you plan to continue on to Confluence Park, retrace your steps to Creekside Landing, turn right, and continue for another 0.6 mile to Confluence Park (see Walk 20). At the park, turn around and return the way you came.

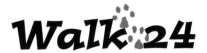

Walk 24

Alamo Placita Park to Speer Gazebo

General location: Cherry Creek area.

Special attractions: A Greenbelt oasis in the middle of a city, occasional raft floats in the creek during high water, well-landscaped streambanks, access to the water. You'll find flower plantings and a gazebo structure in the pocket park at Speer and Lincoln.

Open: 5 A.M. to 11 P.M.

Total distance: 1.8 miles round trip.

Estimated time: 50 minutes to 1¼ hours.

Services: None.

Restrictions: Your dog must be on a leash; pick up after your pet. Keep to the right to permit bicyclists to pass on your left.

For more information: Denver Parks and Recreation Department, (303) 698–4903

Getting started

From I–25, take exit 203 (University Boulevard) and drive north on University to First Avenue (which soon becomes Speer Boulevard). Turn left (west) and drive to Ogden Street. Make a right and park your car on the street.

From downtown Denver at Broadway, head east on Speer Boulevard to Downing Street. Turn left onto the overpass across Cherry Creek. Make another left onto westbound Speer, then turn right onto Ogden and park.

Overview

As it leaves the Cherry Creek Shopping Center area, the Cherry Creek Greenway Trail crosses University Boulevard through an unlit, not particularly pleasant underpass, then follows Speer Boulevard

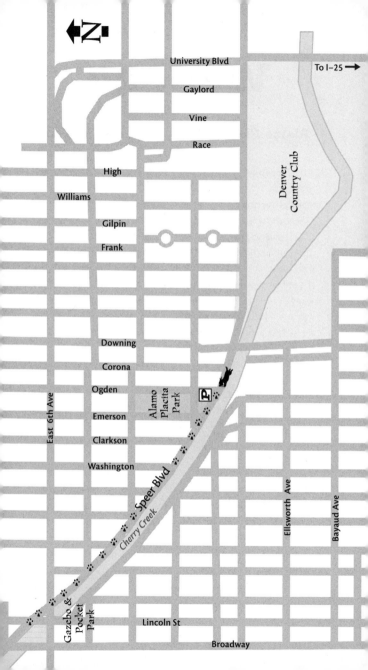

along the sidewalk, while the creek flows through the private Denver
Country Club. The creek and the path are reunited at Downing
Street, where there's access to the path from a ramp between
Downing and Ogden Streets. The path and creek run along a wide,
well-landscaped greenbelt that is, unfortunately, situated between
the east- and westbound lanes of Speer Boulevard, a major street in
Denver. There are nearly a dozen access ramps to the greenbelt,
but all require crossing the westbound lanes of Speer. This walk
begins where there's plentiful side-street parking around the 2-block
Alamo Placita Park. A traffic light enables a safe crossing to the
greenbelt.

This walk is particularly pleasant from June to September, because
Alamo Placita Park is famous for its elaborate and beautiful plantings
of annual flowers.

Since the Cherry Creek Greenway Trail is paved for its entire
length, it's a favorite with bicyclists and in-line skaters. Remember
to keep to the right so that the faster-moving bikers and skaters
can pass you on your left.

The walk

🐾 After leashing your dog, walk 1 block east from Alamo Placita
Park to Downing Street, then carefully cross the westbound lanes of
Speer at the traffic signal. Turn right; the ramp to the greenway and
the creek is immediately on your left.

🐾 At the greenway trail turn right and continue for 0.8 mile to
the overpass at Lincoln Street.

The creek's banks were landscaped during the 1980s and 1990s
and are well maintained. The bank gently slopes down to the water,
and there are many places where you and your pet can dally at the
water's edge. Except for several man-made rapids, the creek flows
gently, and the creekbed is flat and sandy.

🐾 The overpasses are clearly marked with street names. At the
Lincoln Street overpass, take the ramp up to street level. You'll
find yourself in a pocket park in the middle of the intersection of

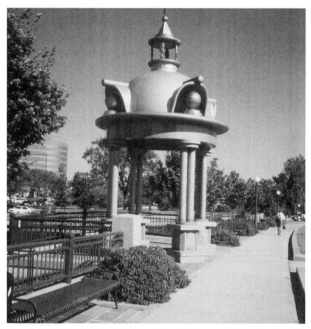

The silver- and gold-domed Speer Gazebo is a prominent landmark on the way to downtown Denver.

four major Denver streets: Sixth Avenue, Lincoln Street, Broadway, and Speer Boulevard. In the early 1990s Speer was diverted into an underpass and the intersection, just short of downtown, was refurbished.

A silver and gold gazebo-type structure dominates the pocket park. There are numerous benches where you can enjoy watching the traffic from an oasis of greenery. The parking lot adjacent to the park serves a Burger King. A McDonald's is across the street on Sixth Avenue. Pedestrian traffic signals connect the park to adjacent streets.

🦴 Turn around and return the way you came.

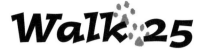

Walk 25

Four Mile House Park

General location: Glendale
and central Denver.

Special attractions: Six parks,
one of them historic.

Open: 5 A.M. to 11 P.M.

Total distance: 4.8 miles round
trip.

Estimated time: 2½ to 3 hours.

Services: Rest rooms, water, picnic tables, and benches.

Restrictions: Your dog must be
on a leash; pick up after your
pet.

For more information: Denver
Parks and Recreation
Department, (303) 698–4903;
Glendale Recreation
Department, (303) 759–1513;
Four Mile Historic Park, (303)
399–1859.

Getting started

This walk through Glendale and east-central Denver can be reached
from several directions.

From Monaco Parkway, take Cherry Creek Drive North past
Garland Park to its intersection with South Holly Street. Parking is
available on the road that curves through Garland Park, you can
park on the wide shoulder on Cherry Creek Drive between Monaco
and Holly. Garland Park has a pond, a sports field, and beautiful
plantings of annual flowers. The flower beds are located at Monaco
Parkway and Cherry Creek Drive.

It's easy to make this outing a shuttle, since there's plentiful
parking at the Cherry Creek Shopping Center, where the walk ends.
To reach the mall, make a right onto Cherry Creek Drive South
from southbound South Holly Street, and continue to Colorado
Boulevard. Turn north (right) onto Colorado, drive 1 block to Cherry
Creek Drive North, and make a left. Continue to the Cherry Creek
Shopping Center and access to parking on your left.

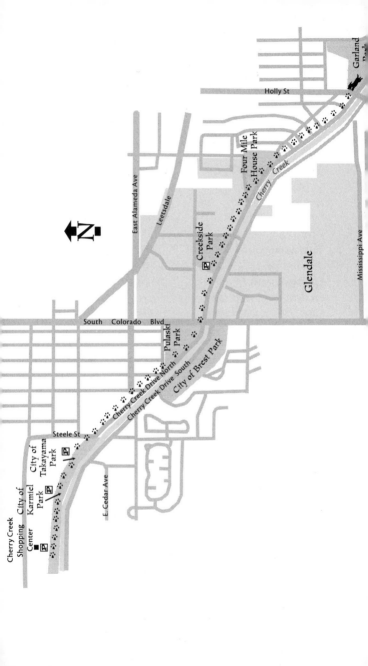

Overview

The Cherry Creek Greenway runs through a portion of Glendale, a small municipality surrounded by Denver, and the trail's location is both a plus and a detriment. The advantage is that the reclaimed and spruced-up creek offers a strip of lush greenery that's not only pleasant for people but also a shelter and habitat for wildlife. On the minus side, traffic noise is never far away. In the stretches where the paved trail runs alongside Cherry Creek Drive South or North, the noise, pollution, and congestion can mitigate your outdoor experience. And crossing busy streets with a pet can be a hazard. Thus, I've chosen for this walk a section of the greenway that's sheltered from the urban experience by six parks and doesn't require surface crossing of busy intersections. You'll pass Four Mile House Park, Creekside Park, Pulaski Park, City of Brest Park, City of Takayama Park, and City of Karmiel Park.

The walk

🦴 After leashing your dog, cross South Holly Street to the Cherry Creek Greenway. You can either use the wide, hard-packed dirt trail or the paved trail. You'll share the paved trail with many bikers and in-line skaters, so stay to your right.

🦴 At 0.6 mile a paved sidewalk to the right serves as a neighborhood access to the greenway. It also marks the beginning of Four Mile House Park, which stretches on your right for 0.2 mile.

Signs along this stretch of the trail explain some of the features of the historic site, which contains the oldest house in Denver, built as an early stagecoach stop. Pets are not allowed in the park; the entrance is at Exposition Street.

🦴 The dirt path ends at Exposition Street as the greenway skirts the street, then continues through an underpass built in 1999 below the busy intersection of Cherry and Exposition Streets. Continue past Creekside Park on your right, where you'll find rest rooms, water, and picnic tables.

🦴 In another 0.6 mile the trail passes under Colorado Boulevard,

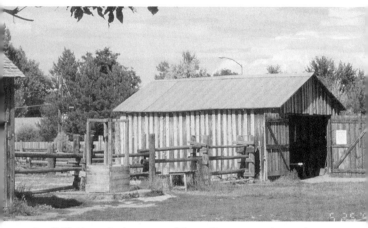

Four Mile House Park was one of the earliest stagecoach stops in Denver.

continues through Pulaski and City of Brest Parks, and curves toward the mall at the Cherry Creek Shopping Center. It divides at the five-level parking structure.

The right fork heads past the shopping center and two restaurants, Chevys and Spinnakers, which have outdoor tables. Your well-behaved dog can join you at an outdoor table for a meal as long as there aren't too many other patrons. This stretch of the trail is dotted with benches.

The left fork of the trail drops to the creek then crosses it on a low bridge that offers your pet easy access to a nice wallow in the sandy, shallow stream.

🦴 The trail then rises to street level and skirts the shopping center's garage as well as a parking lot for the strip mall that extends to University Boulevard.

🦴 Turn around and return the way you came, or, if you decided on a shuttle, pick up your car.

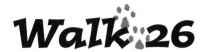

Walk 26

Cherry Creek and High Line Canal Intersection

General location: Denver–
Aurora city limit.

Special attractions: The inter-
section of Cherry Creek
Greenway and the High Line
Canal Trail.

Open: 5 A.M. to 11 P.M.

Total distance: 2.2 miles round
trip.

Estimated time: 1 to 1½ hours.

Services: None.

Restrictions: Your dog must be
on a leash. Pick up after your
pet.

For more information: Denver
Department of Parks and
Recreation, (303) 698–4903.

Getting started

This isn't an easy place to reach, but it's worth the effort to see the
intersection of Cherry Creek and the High Line Canal. From I–25,
take exit 201 (Hampden Avenue) and proceed east for 1.8 miles to
a stoplight at Yosemite. Turn left (north) and proceed for 0.5 mile,
making certain to make a sharp turn right when Yosemite turns to
the right at a fork in the road. Take the first right after this turn,
onto Cornell Avenue. Continue for 5 blocks to Boston Court. Park
on the street. Streets farther down Cornell also dead-end in the
open space and provide on-street parking.

Overview

Where Cherry Creek and the High Line Canal intersect, a large
cement structure channels the two waterways, preventing them
from mingling with each other. The intersection also is one of
two links that the Cherry Creek Greenway provides in the Denver
greenbelt trail system. (The other is with the South Platte River

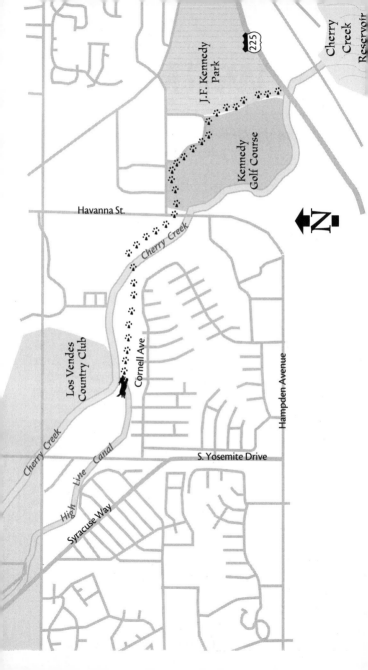

J.F. Kennedy Park

Cherry Creek Reservoir

225

Kennedy Golf Course

Havanna St.

Cherry Creek

N

Los Vendes Country Club

Cornell Ave

Cherry Creek

High Line Canal

Hampden Avenue

S. Yosemite Drive

Syracuse Way

Greenway.) Because two greenbelts intersect here and there are two nearby golf courses, the open space is wide and rolling, and you're all but unaware that I–225 is nearby.

The walk

🐾 After parking your car and putting your dog on a leash, walk straight to the end of Boston Court, which dead-ends in open space. Proceed for a 100 feet or so to a sign that points the way to the High Line Canal Trail and Cherry Creek Greenway. Turn right and walk another 100 or so feet to a raised concrete structure. Here you can see how the flume channels High Line Canal away from Cherry Creek.

🐾 Retrace your steps to the sign and follow the arrow to the Cherry Creek Greenway, which continues in a southeasterly direction across a large meadow. Numerous trails crisscross the meadow and lead to other access streets in the neighborhood. Continue across a bridge over a small creek, and then to a large bridge over Cherry Creek.

Many of the footpaths lead to the creek, where your dog can refresh himself in the shallow water. The John F. Kennedy Golf Course is north and east of Cherry Creek. Ahead is an underpass crossing of Hampden/Havana. Beyond is I–225 and beyond that, the road on top of the Cherry Creek Dam. The rumble of traffic will get louder if you continue, so you may want to turn around and return the way you came.

🐾 If you choose to continue, the trail crosses Hampden/Havana, runs for a block along Dartmouth Avenue, then turns right and continues on Kenton Street between a condo development on your left and the Kennedy Golf Course, which straddles Hampden/Havana, on your right. The trail next runs between the golf course and the J. F. Kennedy Park.

🐾 Beyond the course and the park, the path goes through a low, unlit underpass under I–225, passes three sluices from the dam that eject water into Cherry Creek, then turns east and climbs up to Dam Road before descending into Cherry Creek State Park. There is no shade in this area, and the climb up to the dam is hot and strenuous.

🦴 Turn around and return the way you came.

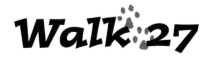

Walk 27

Star K Ranch Open Space

General location: Aurora.

Special attractions: Little-visited open space along Sand Creek.

Open: 5 A.M. to 11 P.M.

Total distance: 2.4 miles round trip.

Estimated time: 40 minutes to 1 hour.

Services: None.

Restrictions: Your dog must be on a leash no longer than 10 feet. Clean up after your pet.

For more information: Aurora Parks and Open Space Department, (303) 739–7160

Getting started

From I–70, take exit 283 (Chambers Road) south. Continue over the railroad tracks to Smith Road. Turn left (east) and drive for 0.6 mile, then turn right (south) onto Laredo Street. This is a narrow dirt road marked by a vertical sign for Emilene's Sirloin House. Continue for 0.1 mile to an AURORA OPEN SPACE marker on the left. Park on the shoulder of the road. The road dead-ends in about 200 feet at the Emilene's parking lot, where there are two conestoga wagons on display. Emilene's is particularly popular with ranchers during the National Western Stock Show.

Overview

The Star K Ranch is a recent (1990s) acquisition by the city of Aurora. Still mostly in its natural state, the open space offers meadows interspersed with stands of cottonwoods. Sand Creek, the most recently designated greenway, flows in a deep gulch south of the walk area. A 5-mile-long trail along Sand Creek from Star K

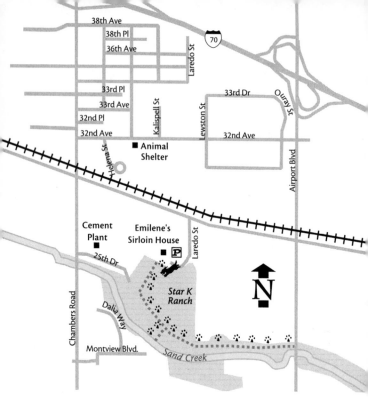

Ranch west to Sand Creek Park at Havana Street and Twenty-sixth
Avenue will be completed in late 2001 (see Walk 28).

The walk

🦴 Pass through the chain at the gate and walk on an improved
crushed-gravel path. There is a bench on the right about 200 feet
from the entry. The gravel trail ends in a rutted jeep road. This trail,
improved in 2000, runs west to Chambers Road and east to Airport
Boulevard. The Chambers Road leg would take you past a working
cement plant, so turn left (east).

🦴 About 0.5 mile into the walk, a stand of tall cottonwoods marks two unimproved footpaths that lead down into the gulch and to Sand Creek.

🦴 The easterly portion of the jeep road continues through a meadow with several giant cottonwood trees to Airport Boulevard. Or, if you would like to descend to Sand Creek, take the unimproved footpath to your right that leads down into a gulch. Follow it to Sand Creek. The ford is shallow, and the sandy bottom here is testament to how the creek got its name. Unless you want to remove your shoes and ford the creek, this is a good place to turn around. It's also an ideal spot for your dog to frolic in the shallow, quiet water. Return the way you came.

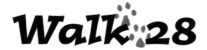

Walk 28

Sand Creek at Bluff Lake

General location: East Denver.
Special attractions: A little-visited trail offering fabulous views of Denver's skyline and the Front Range.
Open: 6 A.M. to 8 P.M.
Total distance: 2 miles round trip to Bluff Lake via Havana; add 0.6 mile for a loop around Bluff Lake.
Estimated time: 40 minutes to 2 hours.

Services: Rest rooms.
Restrictions: Your dog must be on a leash. No pets are allowed on the loop to Bluff Lake.
For more information: Denver Parks and Recreation Department, (303) 698–4903; the Bluff Lake Nature Center, (303) 375–9250.

Getting started

From I-70, take exit 280 (Havana Street) and drive south for 0.5 mile to Smith Road. Turn right (west) and continue on Smith Road for 0.3 mile to an open gate in a chain-link fence. Park in the gravel parking lot inside the fence. Smith Road ends a few hundred feet to the west at the high fence that surrounds the former Stapleton Airport.

Overview

The Sand Creek Greenway became a reality when the Stapleton airport was relocated to Denver International Airport northeast of Denver, because Sand Creek flows through the formerly restricted airport property. In the late 1990s a portion of the greeenway was completed from the edge of the Stapleton property southeast along the creek to Bluff Lake. The reclamation was funded with monies from the Colorado Lottery.

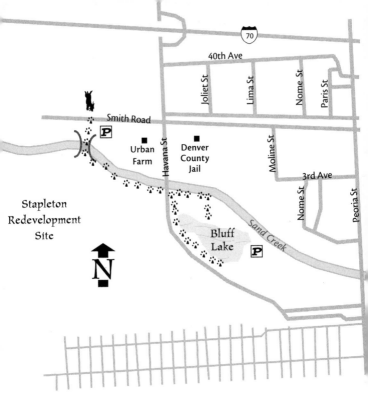

Eventually Sand Creek Park will be constructed at Havana Street and Twenty-Sixth Avenue, and a series of pedestrian bridges will connect it to the Sand Creek Greenway Trail. The construction will connect this portion of the trail with the section east of Chambers Road at Star K Ranch Open Space (see Walk 27).

The Urban Farm Facility, which you'll drive by on Smith Road, provides programs for at-risk inner-city children, who participate in farm-based activities and learn about the environment and agriculture.

A pavilion and rest rooms are located at a high point at Bluff Lake, on Havana Street 0.6 mile south from its intersection with Smith Road. Bluff Lake lies east of the pavilion in a low-lying, marshy gulch. A wide, crushed-gravel trail descends from the pavilion to the lake. Short boardwalks radiating from the trail lead through marshes to two observation points. Pets are not allowed in the vicinity of Bluff Lake, so as not to disturb its rich variety of waterfowl and wild animals. Mosquitoes are a real nuisance in this area.

The walk

🦴 After leashing your dog, pick up the wide, crushed-gravel trail south of the parking lot. In a few hundred feet a high, wide bridge takes you over Sand Creek—more a river than a creek in this vicinity. In the distance to the east, you'll see a small, man-made waterfall over which Sand Creek cascades, drowning out the sound of Havana Street beyond. Walk along the trail for 0.6 mile, swinging south away from Sand Creek at one point, then descending in a curve back to the stream. This portion of the trail is devoid of shade and best hiked early in the morning or in late afternoon. When the trail parallels the creek bank, it's paved. Here are several good spots to stop and give your dog access to the water.

🦴 The trail and creek continue under the Havana Street overpass. At this point you have a choice.

You can follow the trail as it climbs up to Havana Street, where it turns right (south) and becomes a wide sidewalk separated from the road by a wide grassy strip. The trail climbs the bluff, ending at the pavilion above Bluff Lake, where you'll find a large parking lot as well as rest rooms. This route lends itself easily to a shuttle.

🦴 To explore a more interesting trail, turn left (east) onto a clearly visible jeep road and leave the crushed-gravel trail as it climbs to Havana Street. Follow the jeep trail along the bank of Sand Creek. The series of structures across the creek is the Denver County Jail complex. Notice that the banks of Sand Creek have been cleaned of industrial debris, and the channel terraced with large boulders. In addition, cottonwoods and other trees have been planted along the water.

🦴 Continue on the jeep road for another 0.2 mile until it dead-ends in a narrow crushed-gravel trail that runs in both directions. This is part of a series of trails that lead to Bluff Lake and to the pavilion on Havana Street. Since pets are not allowed in the vicinity of Bluff Lake, turn around here. If you're walking without a pet, the gravel path makes a 0.2-mile loop. Halfway around the loop, a boardwalk leads through tall cattails to an overlook of the lake. There's also a toilet and a bench on the loop. Mosquitoes can be fierce in this area. Return the way you came.

The Foothills

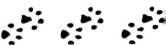

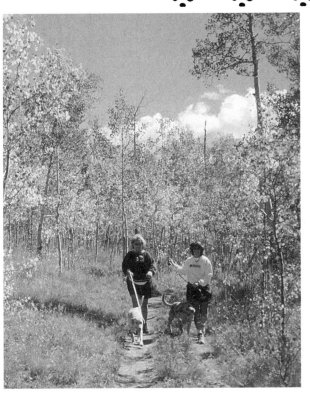

The Foothills

The strip of land where the Great Plains meet the Rocky Mountains offers some of the most magnificent scenery anywhere. Rolling grasslands end in craggy rock formations or are uplifted to become pine-covered foothills. Beyond the hills rise rugged peaks carved by erosion and mountain streams that tumble to the prairie.

The Arapahoe once inhabited this land, while the Ute tribe controlled the inner mountains. Maj. Stephen Long—for whom Longs Peak is named—explored the Front Range and foothills in 1820. Although he found the scenery arresting, he dismissed the undulating prairie as the "Great American Desert."

Settlers came following Lewis Ralston's 1850 discovery of gold in a tributary of Clear Creek. A second gold strike in 1858 near the confluence of Cherry Creek and the South Platte River led to the establishment of Denver and set off what came to be known as the Pike's Peak Gold Rush.

As more gold was discovered in the mountains, towns sprang up along the mouths of the canyons that led through the foothills into the interior. Mount Vernon, founded by a gold-seeking preacher, was built at the entrance to Mount Vernon canyon—the present-day route of I–70. Just to the north, Apex City arose at the mouth of Amos (now Apex) Gulch and is today's Heritage Square. Golden City, which would become the home of Coors Beer in 1880, was founded at the entrance to Clear Creek canyon. Golden Gate City, which gave its name to Golden Gate State Park, was built at the entrance to Tucker Gulch, while Morrison arose at the point where Bear Creek exits the mountains.

Denver began acquiring land in the mountains and the foothills in 1878 to gain control of the precious water in the South Platte River and other waterways. However, local efforts to preserve the craggy formations, the rolling grasslands, and access to mountain streams did not gain momentum until the second half of the twentieth century. Both Boulder and Jefferson Counties established open-space acquisition programs in 1972. Bear Creek Lake Park came into existence when the Bear Creek Dam was completed in 1982.

As Denver, its suburbs, and its satellite towns continue to grow, the open spaces are where we go to seek solitude or to hike with our pet striding quietly at our side. Rock Creek Farm, on the easternmost boundary of Boulder County Open Space, is a remarkable refuge from the bustle and noise of urban life—literally across the road from it. Bear Creek Lake Park preserves a riparian environment, as does Jefferson County Open Space's Lair o' the Bear Park. The Matthew-Winters Open Space Park not only encompasses the old ghost town of Mount Vernon but also gives you the opportunity to hike in the shadow of the red rocks of the Fountain Formation—the flame-red remnant of the original Rocky Mountains. Only by walking these areas can you truly enjoy the strip of land where prairie and mountains meet.

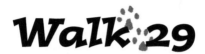

Walk 29

Rock Creek Farm

General location: Louisville/
Broomfield.

Special attractions: A working
farm and sweeping views of
the prairie and the Front
Range.

Open: Sunrise to sunset.

Total distance: 1.5 miles round
trip.

Estimated time: 1 to 1½ hours.

Services: Rest rooms, picnic
tables, and interpretive signs
at the South 104th Street
parking lot only.

Restrictions: Your dog must be
on a leash.

For more information:
Boulder County Parks and
Open Space, (303) 441–3950.

Getting started

Take U.S. 36 west to the U.S. 287/Broomfield/Lafayette exit. Drive
north on U.S. 287 for 2.9 miles to a stoplight at Dillon Road. Turn
left (west), drive 0.8 mile, and make a left (south) onto South 104th
Street. Drive 0.7 mile to the parking lot.

Overview

Walking Rock Creek Farm is like being in Colorado 150 years ago.
This open space embodies the tranquility of the open prairie before
settlement and urbanization.

Rock Creek Farm lies at the easternmost edge of the Boulder
County Open Space, across U.S. 287 from booming Broomfield
County. Yet once you're a few hundred yards into the walk, you're
alone. To the west, the Rockies rise into the dome of the sky, and
the vistas are wide and unobstructed.

First inhabited by Indians, the land became a farm during the
1859 gold rush. Mary and Lafayette Miller, founders of the nearby

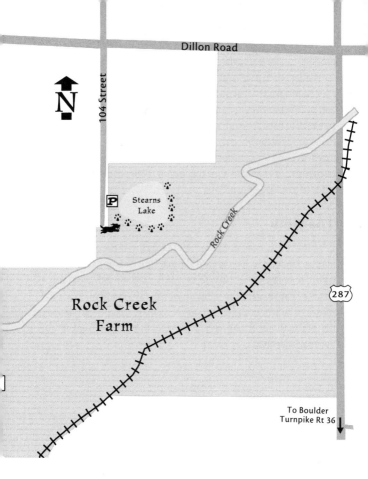

town of Lafayette, purchased eighty acres here that included the Overland Mail Stage Route stop used by the Pony Express in 1870. Later Abner C. Goodhue, founder of the Goodhue Ditch and Reservoir Company, operated a horse and cattle ranch on the property until 1924. Crop raising and ranching have continued on the property to the present.

Boulder County purchased the 994-acre farm in 1980 as part of its greenbelt and urban buffer. The county leases part of the property to tenant farmers who raise corn and other crops, while remainder is grassland and wildlife habitat.

Stearns Lake attracts herons, cormorants, and grebes; its northern and northwestern portions, which are swampy, have been set aside as a wildlife habitat. South of the lake Rock Creek creates a greenbelt marked by cottonwoods, chokecherries, and willows. In 2000 Rock Creek received a grant from Colorado Lottery funds. This money is being used to eliminate a parking lot on Dillon Road and to create a future trail along Rock Creek.

The walk

After leashing your dog, find the trailhead on the southeast side of the parking lot. Proceed through the gate onto a wide, flat trail that circles Stearn Lake. Continue east then north around the lake, looking for signs that indicate whether the wildlife area on the west and north sides of the lake is open. If so, you can explore the north shore of the lake. Otherwise, turn around and return the way you came.

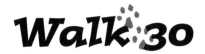

Walk 30

Bear Creek Lake Park

General location: Lakewood.

Special attractions: A large reservoir whose diverse habitats range from prairie to lakefront and canyon.

Open: 5:00 A.M. to 11:00 P.M.

Total distance: 1.7 miles round trip.

Estimated time: 40 minutes to 1 hour.

Services: Portable toilets, picnic tables.

Restrictions: A daily entrance fee of $4 is required. You must keep your pet on a leash and pick up after him.

For more information: City of Lakewood, (303) 697–6159 or 697–8190.

Getting started

Take the Morrison Road exit off C–470. Drive east on Morrison Road for 0.1 mile to the Bear Creek Lake Park entrance on your right. After paying your fee at the entrance booth, proceed to a stop sign. Bear left and drive to the second parking lot on your right (south side of the road). There's a portable toilet; farther on are several picnic tables.

Overview

At roughly 2,500 acres, Bear Creek Lake Park is the city of Lakewood's largest park. It's open year-round and, in addition to trails around the reservoir and along Bear Creek, offers fishing, boating, camping, boat rentals, a water ski school, and equestrian and biking trails. With its diversity of habitats, the park features a wide variety of plant and wildlife species, making a walk here particularly interesting. Besides the commonly found prairie dogs, deer, and coyotes, Bear Creek Lake Park has also attracted occasional elk, mountain lions, and migrating bald eagles.

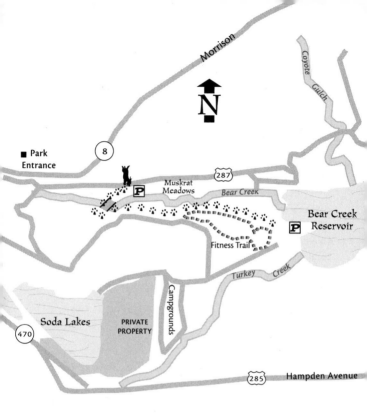

The park has 5.5 miles of paved trails and 15 miles of soft-surface trails. The walk described here is a shady, pleasant jaunt along Bear Creek and through stands of tall cottonwoods and thick underbrush watered by the stream. Part of the walk follows a fitness trail that leads to a large parking lot overlooking Bear Creek Lake.

The walk

After putting your pet on a leash, walk south from the parking lot to Bear Creek, then turn right (west) and follow the creekside horse trail to a footbridge. Cross the creek, turn left (east), and follow the horse trail downstream.

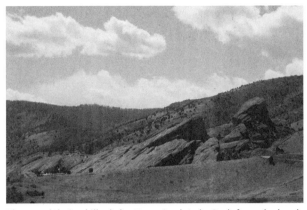

These undulating hills shelter Bear Creek Lake Park from the bustle of the metro area.

At an intersection with the fitness trail, note the fitness stations on both the right and left sides of the pathway. Leave the horse trail and proceed straight ahead on the fitness trail until you reach the first station. You'll find yourself in a large dirt parking lot. Cross it to reach the lake. This area is called Pelican Point. The shoreline is sandy and slopes gently, so that your pet can have a refreshing wallow. Turn around and return the way you came.

You can also return by following the southerly loop of the fitness trail to the point where it intersects with the horse trail. This segment skirts the road to the lake, however, and is not as pleasant as the shaded northerly trail.

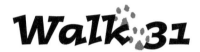

Walk 31

Standley Lake Regional Park (South)

General location: Arvada and Westminster.

Special attractions: A large lake, and a large meadow that has been preserved as a prairie.

Open: 8:00 A.M. to 8:00 P.M.

Total distance: Loop, 1 mile; east loop, 2 miles.

Estimated time: 50 minutes to 1 hour for each loop.

Services: Portable toilets, covered picnic areas.

Restrictions: Your dog must be on a leash. Pets are not permited to swim in the reservoir.

For more information:
Standley Lake Regional Park Office, (303) 425–1097.

Getting started

Take I–70 to exit 269 (Wadsworth Boulevard) and proceed north on Wadsworth for 3.7 miles to West Eightieth Avenue. Turn left (west) and continue to Kipling Street. Turn right (north) and proceed until Kipling dead-ends at West Eighty-sixth Parkway. Turn left (west) and drive 1 mile to the park entrance, on your right. The entrance comes up quickly, so keep an eye out for it. It's across from Simms Street.

Overview

This is a lovely 3,000-acre grassland area in the northwestern suburbs, with sweeping views to the Flatirons and Longs Peak to the northwest. Although many reservoirs in the Denver area are surrounded by marinas, parking lots, and mowed expanses of grass, Standley Lake is a notable exception. The park is preserved as a natural prairie that stretches for 2 miles on both north and south lakeshores and acts as a buffer between homes and the lake.

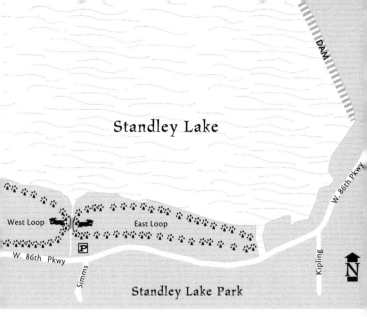

On a blustery day, the shore is reminiscent of the Maine coast. The wind sweeps down from the mountains and whips the lake into whitecaps, while screaming gulls soar on the air currents or swoop down to fish. The reservoir is the water source for the cities of Westminster, Northglenn, and Thornton, so neither you nor your pet can swim here. The lake is used for boating and fishing and is stocked with trout, bass, catfish, and perch.

Two gazebolike structures with picnic tables are perched on the upper trail and offer panoramic views.

Since the dirt parking lot is in the middle of the open space, you can walk either right or left. Both loops have an upper and lower trail that join at the parking lot and again at the inlets on either end of the lake. The right (east) loop is a little longer.

The walk

West Loop: After leashing your dog, walk north from the parking lot on a broad trail. Cross a bridge over a creek and turn left. At the fork turn left (south) and take the broad, jeeplike trail west for 0.6 mile to an inlet at the end of the open space. A sign marks the park boundary. Turn right (north) and continue to the lakeshore, then follow the shore trail back to your starting point.

East Loop: After putting your dog on a leash, walk north from the parking lot on a broad trail. Cross a bridge over a creek and turn right (east). At the fork turn right (south) and take the broad, jeeplike trail east for 1 mile to an inlet at the end of the open space. Turn left (north) and continue to the lakeshore, then follow the shore trail back to your starting point.

Several trails crisscross the grassland; the two most popular lead to two gazebolike picnic tables that offer panoramic views of the lake and the Front Range (see Walk 32).

Walk 32
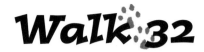

Standley Lake Regional Park (North)

General location: Westminster.

Special attractions: A large lake, and large meadows that have been preserved as prairie. There's a nearby bald eagle wildlife area.

Open: Sunrise to sunset.

Total distance: 2-mile loop.

Estimated time: 40 to 50 minutes.

Services: Rest rooms and covered picnic areas.

Restrictions: Your dog must be on a leash. Pets are not permitted to swim in the reservoir.

For more information: Standley Lake Regional Park Office, (303) 425–1097.

Getting started

Take U.S. 36, the Boulder Turnpike, to the Church Ranch Boulevard exit, then follow Church Ranch Boulevard southwest to Wadsworth Boulevard. After crossing Wadsworth, the road name changes to East Hundredth Avenue. Proceed for about a mile. The park will open on your left. Look for the intersection with Owens Street; right across from this intersection is a dirt parking lot, where you can leave your vehicle. This lot allows you to access the park without paying the entry fee. If you plan to fish or boat, drive farther west to Simms Street, where you'll find a park entrance on your left. Drive to the entry booth. The day charge is $5. Continue to the large parking lot by the lake.

Overview

This lovely grassland area in the northwestern suburbs features sweeping views of the mountains and a unique bald eagle sanctuary, operated by Jefferson County Open Space, in the northwest corner

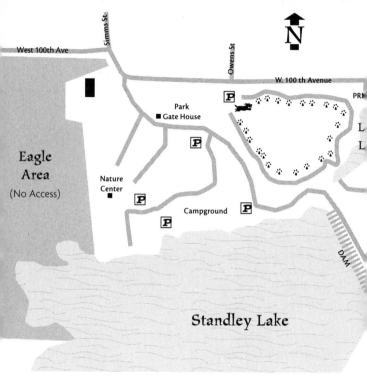

of the park. Although there are eagle viewing areas, the sanctuary is not open to the public.

A pair of bald eagles built a nest in 1992 in the stand of cottonwoods in this area. The pair has returned annually to breed. Despite its 3,000-acre size, the Standley Lake Park is considered "urban" for bald eagles. However, the plentiful fish in the lake and the park's many prairie dog colonies offer the birds a sustaining habitat.

The walk

From the parking lot across from Owens Street, walk left (east) on a broad, soft-surface trail. You'll hear the chatter of prairie dogs all over the meadow you're crossing. Proceed on the trail until

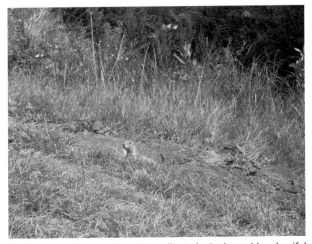

The large prairie dog colony at Standley Lake Park provides plentiful food for bald eagles nesting in the nearby bird sanctuary.

it approaches Loon Lake, which marks the eastern boundary of the park and is privately held.

🦴 Pass the lake and look for a rugged jeep road on your right. This road parallels a usually dry gulch that runs west from Loon Lake; follow it westward. As you approach a stand of cottonwoods, you'll see the parking lot where you left your car. Turn right onto a narrow trail that leads back to your vehicle.

Other walks are possible here. You might want to explore the lakeshore, where there are usually several anglers in search of bass, trout, and other fish that are stocked annually (see also Walk 31). Your dog cannot enter the lake, however, because it's used as a potable water supply. Swimming is not allowed.

Walk 33

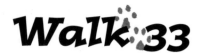

Van Bibber Park

General location: Arvada.

Special attractions: Beautiful views, urban open space, and a stream.

Open: One hour before sunrise to one hour after sunset.

Total distance: 3 miles round trip.

Estimated time: 40 minutes to 1 hour.

Services: Rest rooms and water fountains at the Ward Road parking lot.

Restrictions: Your dog must be on a leash. Pick up after your pet.

For more information: Jefferson County Open Space, (303) 271–5925.

Getting started

From I–70 take exit 266 (Ward Road). Drive north for 1.1 miles to the park entrance on your left. Ward Road is a busy north–south thoroughfare, so turning across two lanes of traffic may be daunting. If you miss the turnoff, which is in the middle of a long stretch of empty land, continue to Fifty-eighth Avenue and turn left (west). Proceed 1.4 miles to Indiana Street. Turn left (south) and drive 0.3 mile; the park's second parking lot is on your left. The walk lends itself to a shuttle.

Overview

An unencumbered view of the foothills is what's great about this walk, which takes you across a very large grassland that has been left in its natural state. You'll travel the 10-foot-wide concrete Van Bibber Creek Trail, which is wheelchair accessible and also great if you're taking along a child in a stroller. The trail parallels Van Bibber

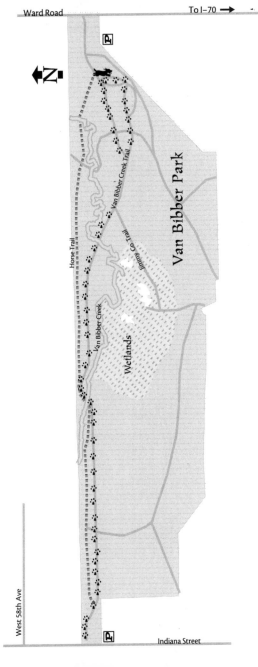

Creek, which runs from west to east across the grassland.

Van Bibber Park is rich with historical connections. In 1850 the first recorded gold strike in Colorado was made nearby on Ralston Creek. This preceded the more famous gold strikes on Cherry Creek. At about the same time, homesteaders began moving into the area, settling on land near the creeks and small lakes that dot the region. Others dug irrigation ditches to divert water to irrigate their crops of wheat, corn, hay, and, later, strawberries. By 1870 there were some 500 residents in the agricultural community, named Arvada. The Ralston Creek Stage Road ran nearby and connected Denver with Boulder and Central City.

A dirt trail that runs diagonally south from the Van Bibber Creek Trail is known as the Jimmy Go Trail, after one of the prior owners of the park property.

The walk

After parking your car and leashing your dog, walk to the edge of either parking lot to pick up the Van Bibber Creek Trail. Walking west from Ward Road is more interesting because of the panoramic view of the mountains, but you can walk this 1.5-mile trail from either lot. If you'd rather not walk on concrete, take one of the many dirt side trails to a 4-foot-wide horse trail that parallels the concrete path. The horse trail is situated about 100 feet north of the concrete path.

About 1 mile from Ward Road (0.5 mile from Indiana Street), the trail crosses Van Bibber Creek. Here two stands of tall cottonwoods offer shade and access to the water for your pet. Picnic tables under the trees provide a place for a snack or lunch.

Turn around and return the way you came—or, if you've chosen a shuttle walk, pick up your vehicle.

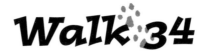

Walk 34

Crown Hill Lake Open Space Park

General location: Wheat Ridge/
Lakewood.

Special attractions: The lake
and panoramic vistas.

Open: One hour before sunrise
to one hour after sunset.

Total distance: Inner loop, 1.2
miles; outer loop, 2 miles.

Estimated time: 1 to 1½ hours.

Services: Rest rooms, picnic
tables, and telephones.

Restrictions: Your dog must be
on a leash.

For more information:
Jefferson County Open Space,
(303) 271–5925.

Getting started

From I–70 take exit 287 (Kipling Street) and drive 2 miles south to
West Twenty-sixth Avenue. Turn left (east) on Twenty-sixth Avenue.
You can either use the small parking lot immediately on your left or
continue to the larger lot 2 blocks farther down the street.

Overview

Crown Hill Lake Open Space Park is located on the boundary
between Wheat Ridge and Lakewood. It was created in 1979,
through the joint efforts of Jefferson County and the cities of Wheat
Ridge and Lakewood. The northwest corner of the park is set aside
as a wildlife sanctuary, dedicated a national urban wildlife refuge by
the National Urban Institute on Earth Day 1991.

The 177-acre park has been kept in a natural state, with minimal
development and an emphasis on preserving habitat for wildlife. The
sanctuary and the lake are home to a variety of wildlife, including
numerous species of waterfowl and shorebirds as well as foxes and
even deer. Approximately 6.5 miles of trails are available. The
primary trail is a paved walkway around the lake. An outer loop

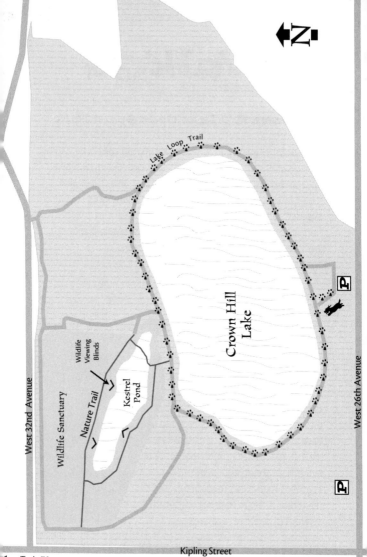

N

Crown Hill Lake

Lake Loop Trail

Wildlife Sanctuary

Wildlife Viewing Blinds

Nature Trail

Kestrel Pond

West 32nd Avenue

West 26th Avenue

Kipling Street

← To I-70

trail follows the park perimeter, but it's rather noisy since it runs along West Thirty-second Avenue and Kipling Street, both busy thoroughfares.

The walk

🦴 Park in either of the parking lots off West Twenty-sixth Avenue. After putting your dog on a leash, proceed past the rest rooms to the paved trail. Turn left (west) and hike along the perimeter of the lake. Watch out for the occasional in-line skater.

There are benches at regular intervals around the loop. The north side of the lake offers several places where you can stop to let your dog get his paws wet. On the eastern portion of the loop, you'll be facing a panorama of the foothills and the distant Front Range.

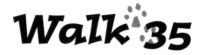

Walk 35

Matthew-Winters Park

General location: Morrison.

Special attractions: Remains of the Mount Vernon ghost town, views of red rocks, and the Red Rocks Amphitheater.

Open: One hour before sunrise to one hour after sunset.

Total distance: This is a 1-mile loop.

Estimated time: 30 minutes.

Services: Rest rooms, water, and picnic tables.

Restrictions: Your dog must be on a leash.

For more information: Jefferson County Open Space, (303) 271–5925.

Getting started

From I–70, take exit 259 (Morrison). At the stoplight at the bottom of the ramp, bear left (south) onto C–26. Continue under the interstate to the park entrance on your right (west). The parking lot offers access both to trails and to the Mount Vernon town site.

Overview

Matthews-Winters Park is located at a major entrance to the Rocky Mountains. The park lies astride the entrance to Mount Vernon canyon, which was one of the early routes to the gold fields of Central City and Fairplay in South Park. Dr. Joseph Casto, a lay preacher and land promoter who came from Ohio to make his fortune during the gold rush, founded the town of Mount Vernon in 1859. He reportedly grubstaked John H. Gregory on his prospect in Gregory Gulch, and is credited with discovering the famous Casto lode near Central City. Casto hoped Mount Vernon would become a supply town along the mining route, so he gave away building

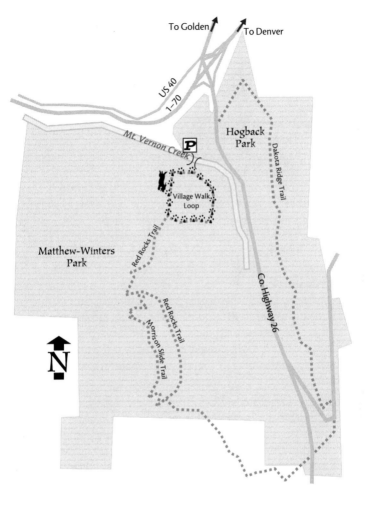

lots at no cost to those who would build on them. By January 1860 Mount Vernon had forty-four registered voters.

Though short lived, the town played an important role in Colorado's formation. It became for a brief time the capital of Jefferson Territory, the name Colorado was first known by. Mount Vernon's fortunes, like those of other boomtowns, waxed and waned under the impact of the Civil War, periodic droughts, floods, Indian raids, and depressions. Although the Mount Vernon route was in continuous use, the town lost out in the struggle to survive as a city.

Today the features that attracted settlers to this spot are still evident to the park visitor. The Dakota Hogback forms a low, rounded barrier between the prairie and the foothills. The park offers a variety of trails. Some climb west up the slopes of the first row of peaks and offer sweeping vistas of the plains beyond the Hogback. In a narrow valley Mount Vernon Creek winds its way through clumps of willows, chokecherries, and wild plums.

The walk described here—a loop not usually frequented by bikers—takes you through the old Mount Vernon town site.

The walk

After parking your car and leashing your dog, head south down the wooden steps from the parking lot to Mount Vernon Creek. Cross the creek and proceed for 0.3 mile uphill. Although the hillside looks like scrub grassland, it's covered by yuccas and prickly pear cactuses, so don't let your dog stray off the well-maintained trail.

At 0.3 mile, the Red Rocks Trail, a favorite of bikers, continues uphill and to the southwest, while the Village Walk Loop turns left (east). You now enter the Mount Vernon town site. Look for an old cemetery where graves date back to the 1860s. Complete the 0.6-mile west arm of the loop and return to the parking area.

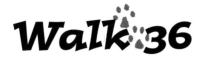

Walk 36

Apex Trail

General location: Golden.

Special attractions: Isolation despite your nearness to civilization. This is an excellent conditioning hike in spring.

Open: One hour before sunrise to one hour after sunset.

Total distance: 5.6 miles round trip.

Estimated time: 3 to 4 hours.

Services: Portable toilets in the parking lot.

Restrictions: Your dog must be on a leash.

For more information:
Jefferson County Open Space, (303) 271–5925.

Getting started

From I–70, take exit 259 (Morrison). At the stoplight at the bottom of the ramp, bear right (north) onto U.S. 40. Continue for 1 mile to the entrance to Heritage Square on your left. Turn into the drive that leads to this shopping mall, then turn right (north) into the lower parking lot. Drive to the northwest corner of the lot, where a large brown-and-beige JEFFERSON COUNTY OPEN SPACE sign marks the trailhead. A portable toilet hidden by a wooden stockade is nearby.

The Apex Trail connects with the Jefferson Nature Center near the summit of Lookout Mountain, so it lends itself well to a shuttle if you want to take only a shorter, one-way hike, either up or down. To reach the northwest end of the trail, drive west on I–70 and take exit 256, (Lookout Mountain). At the top of the ramp, turn left (west) onto the service road. After 1.5 miles turn right (north) onto Lookout Mountain Road. Drive another 1.5 miles to a sign that tells you the nature center is to your left. Park just short of the sign. The shoulder on both sides of the road is wide enough to accommodate

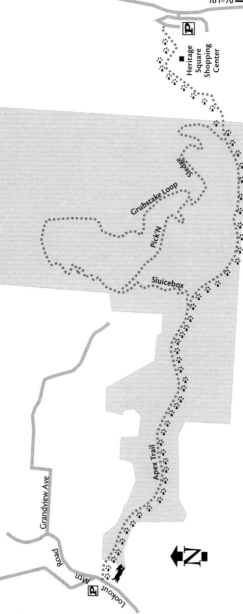

US 40

To I–70 →

P

Heritage
Square
Shopping
Center

Sledge

Grubstake Loop

Pick'N

Sluicebox

Apex Trail

Grandview Ave

Road

Lookout Mtn

P

N

several cars. The trailhead to the Apex Trail is about 30 feet south of the sign and clearly marked.

Overview

Located in the foothills above Golden, the Apex Trail is one in a network of trails that climb the east face of Lookout Mountain. The relatively low altitude makes this a great conditioning hike in spring, when similar trails at higher elevations are still snowbound. It can also help you gauge whether you and your pet are ready for hiking in the mountains. The 1,000-foot elevation gain and rocky terrain make an excellent test of your and your pet's stamina.

During the Colorado gold rush, this trail was a toll road known as the Gregory Wagon Trail. The road connected the frontier settlement Apex—where the present-day Heritage Square Shopping Center is located—with Gregory Diggings, which would become Central City. Tolls were collected in Apex from miners and provisioners headed for the gold fields. There were stables where tired horses could rest; extra teams might be hooked up for the steep uphill haul. Weary travelers could refresh themselves as well at a local inn.

Today signs along the trail recall its past. One announces that the owner of a wagon drawn by a single team of horses, mules, or oxen had to pay a sixty-cent toll, while one cent was charged for every head of sheep passing along the trail.

The present-day hiking trail is narrow, steep, and rocky in many places. It follows Apex Gulch and a creek that offers many opportunities for you to stop and let your pet frolic for a few minutes in the shallow water.

The trail is also used by bikers, who have a job cut out for them negotiating the boulders and the ever-upward climb. On weekdays or when the trail is still snowy or muddy, however, you and your pet will enjoy relative solitude.

The walk

From the lower Heritage Square parking lot, leash your dog and begin hiking west on a dirt trail. As you come upon the upper parking lot, the dirt trail joins a concrete bike path that continues northwest into a subdivision. Cross the creek on a footbridge, then turn west (left) and continue past Heritage Square, where the trail is again packed dirt.

Climb up the gulch, steadily gaining elevation. Several other trails spur off the Apex Trail as it climbs higher; junctions are clearly marked. The Apex Trail follows the creek, which flows to your left. Although the banks of the creek are steep at times, the trail also swoops down to the water at numerous places and the bank becomes flat, making the streambed accessible.

The final 0.25 mile of the trail is an easement that passes among houses. Turn around and return the way you came or, if you opted for a shuttle, retrieve your vehicle.

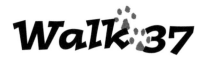

Walk 37

Lair o' the Bear Park

General location: West of Morrison.

Special attractions: A creekside environment in the mountains.

Open: One hour before sunrise to one hour after sunset.

Total distance: 2.4 miles round trip.

Estimated time: 1 to 1½ hours.

Services: Rest rooms, water pump, picnic tables, and benches.

Restrictions: Your dog must be on a leash. Pets are not permitted on the south side of the creek in the Creekside Nature Walk.

For more information: Jefferson County Open Space, (303) 271–5925

Getting started

Take the Morrison Road exit off C–470 and drive west on Morrison through the town of Morrison. Note the bakery on your right at the edge of town. In good weather tables are set outside, and a well-behaved pet can join you while you have a drink, sample the bakery's famous sticky buns, or buy a scoop of homemade ice cream.

Beyond Morrison, bear right onto C–74 toward Evergreen. In 4.5 miles look for the LAIR O' THE BEAR park sign on the left (south) side of the road. The entrance road slopes down from C–74 to a parking lot; it's easy to miss if you're not watchful.

Overview

This open-space park possesses a unique variety of ecological, geological, and scenic features. Geological forces together with erosion formed Bear Creek canyon, and nearly 1.5 miles of Bear

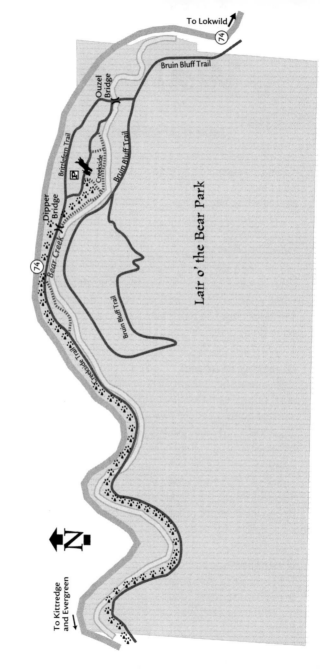

To Lokwild

74

Bruin Bluff Trail

Ouzel
Bridge

Brittlefern Trail

Creekside

Bruin Bluff Trail

P

Dipper
Bridge

Bear Creek

74

Lair o' the Bear Park

Bruin Bluff Trail

Creekside Trail

N

To Kittredge
and Evergreen

Creek lie within the park. The riparian zone along the creek hosts a diversity of plant and animal species. The park is inhabited or visited by deer, elk, small mammals, and birds, as well as by reptiles, amphibians, and waterfowl. Anglers can try their luck with several species, including rainbow and brown trout.

One of the most interesting birds residing in the riparian zone is a small, grayish, wrenlike bird called the American dipper or water ouzel. Children as well as adults love watching these animated birds hopping and bobbing among the rocks along the stream, then suddenly plunging into the water for a meal. Dippers are rather remarkable in that they actually walk along the bottom of the stream, seemingly oblivious to the current, as they feed on insect larvae.

On a fine weekend afternoon, the park is filled with families, children, and pets. The trail described here is upstream along Bear Creek's northern bank. Climbing Bruin Bluff on the south side of the creek is not recommended, because the top of the bluff is narrow and gravelly, with a sheer drop-off of several hundred feet on one side.

The walk

🐾 After putting your dog on a leash, walk south past the JEFFERSON COUNTY OPEN SPACE sign to Bear Creek. A series of concrete steps leads down to the stream. They're wide enough for your dog to use them to reach the water.

🐾 The Creekside Trail runs along the north bank of Bear Creek. Turn right (upstream) and follow the trail.

It will soon enter the shade of tall cottonwoods. The bank levels off to give you and your dog plenty of opportunities to stop and get paws wet. There are also several spots where you can sit at a picnic table or on a bench overlooking the creek. The trail traverses a fertile floodplain that features narrowleaf and plains cottonwoods, alders, chokecherries, and occasional box elders, as well as many stands of willows.

🦴 At 0.2 mile and again at 0.5 mile, you'll pass bridges over Bear Creek that lead to the Creekside Nature Walk. Signs warn that pets are not permitted in the protected area. Continue on the trail upstream.

As you walk farther, the floodplain constricts and the canyon narrows. The moist, rocky surface of the north-facing canyon wall supports a lush array of wildflowers, ferns, and mosses, as well as blue spruce and Douglas fir trees.

🦴 About two-thirds of the way into your hike, the trail crosses the creek on a bridge.

Notice the changes in types of vegetation. South-facing slopes are covered by open stands of ponderosa pine, juniper, yucca, and other plants typical of warm, arid conditions.

🦴 At 1 mile you'll approach the Highway 74 overpass high above the creek. The park ends at the curve in the road. Turn around and return the way you came.

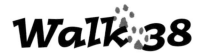

Walk 38

Frazer Meadow

General location: Golden.

Special attractions: Forest environment, meadows, and distant views of the peaks.

Open: The visitor's center is open 6 A.M. to 4 P.M. Overnite camping is allowed by permit.

Total distance: 3.6 miles round trip.

Estimated time: 2½ to 3 hours.

Services: Toilets at the trailhead; rest rooms and water at the visitors center.

Restrictions: Registration at the visitors center is required. Your dog must be on a leash.

For more information: Golden Gate Canyon State Park, (303) 582–3707.

Getting started

The park is located northwest of Golden. Take the Sixth Avenue Freeway, which becomes U.S. 6, to Golden. Drive for 3.5 miles on U.S. 6 to its intersection with C–93 and C–58. U.S. 6 turns west to Black Hawk and Central City; don't go that way. Instead, continue straight ahead (north) on C–93 toward Boulder. In 1 mile look for a sign for GOLDEN GATE STATE PARK. Turn left (west) onto a park access road and drive into the foothills for 13 miles on the twisting, climbing paved road. Once you reach the park, turn right and continue to the visitors center on your right.

If you don't have an annual state park pass, purchase one here. The fee is $4 for a day pass, and $40 for an annual pass. Water, rest rooms, and exhibits of local fauna and flora are found at the center, as well as detailed maps of the park and its environs.

Exit the visitors center parking lot, turn right, and drive for 0.4 mile to the Frazer Meadow Trailhead parking lot on the left. There are toilets here.

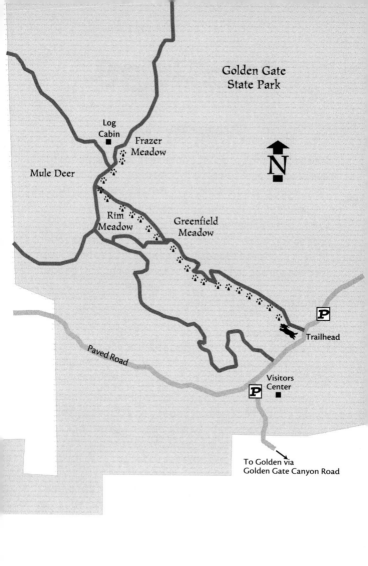

Golden Gate
State Park

Log
Cabin

Frazer
Meadow

Mule Deer

Rim
Meadow

Greenfield
Meadow

N

Paved Road

P

Trailhead

Visitors
Center

P

To Golden via
Golden Gate Canyon Road

Overview

Only 30 miles from Denver, Golden Gate Canyon State Park offers 14,000 acres of conifer forest, rocky peaks, mountain splendor, and aspen-filled meadows. Several ponds offer good trout fishing.

There are twelve trails in the park, each named for an animal and marked with the animal's footprint. The shape of the marker indicates the difficulty of the trail: Circles denote easy trails, squares are moderate, and diamonds mark the difficult trails. Trailheads with parking areas are easily accessible from the main roads in the park.

Golden Gate Canyon State Park takes its name from Golden Gate City, once located at the mouth of Tucker Gulch, which led to the gold fields of Black Hawk and Central City. The two former mining towns, now popular as limited-stakes gambling destinations, are 6 miles south of the park on C–119. Despite the coming of gambling casinos, these towns continue to offer a glimpse of life in Colorado's early days.

The walk

🐾 After putting your dog on a leash, head to the Frazer Meadow Trailhead. Hike on the well-maintained trail, following and crossing Ralston Creek five times on sturdy footbridges. You're on the Horseshoe Trail, which is clearly and frequently marked with the sign of a horseshoe.

🐾 Cross a bridge and continue slowly climbing the aspen-covered hillside. Cross the creek again, and then for a third time.

You're traveling through stands of aspen, which makes this hike particularly pleasant in September when the trees change color. Eventually the trees begin to thin, and you pass through several small meadows.

🐾 About halfway to Frazer Meadow, look for a sign pointing to the Greenfield Meadow and Rim Meadow Campsites. Black Bear Trail heads off to the left. At this junction you're about halfway to Frazer Meadow.

Continue on the Horseshoe Trail. The next creek crossing is flat and sandy, offering a good place to stop and let your dog take a quick dip in the creek.

The trail becomes steep and switchbacks several times, crossing the creek twice more. The fifth footbridge offers another easy access to the water for your pet. Stay on Horseshoe Trail when it merges with the Mule Deer Trail. There's a clear sign pointing to Frazer Meadow to your right. Continue another 0.1 mile to reach this large, open meadow.

There's a ruined cabin to explore on the edge of Frazer Meadow. Tremont Mountain rises to the north, and a broad view extends southward through the valley. Sit on a downed log and take in the scenery. The meadow is also famous for its early-spring wild irises.

🦴 Turn around and return the way you came.

Dog Heavens

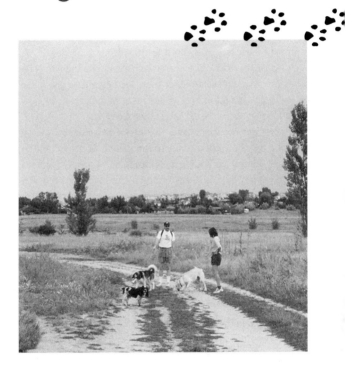

Dog Heavens

To leash or not to leash? Perhaps the most controversial issue concerning pets in the urban environment is leash laws. The most often-heard argument against these laws is that a dog cannot be properly exercised when on a leash. Indeed, some dog lovers have tried to get around the leash requirement by using retracting leashes that may extend for 15 or more feet, essentially giving the dog free reign. As a result, Denver and other municipalities are now mandating that leashes be no longer than 6 feet.

Yet most park personnel and open-space rangers acknowledge that a dog needs the opportunity to run free, to be trained, and to learn voice control. To answer these needs, some areas have been set aside for dog training. Here a dog can run off leash safely and legally. As of this writing, there are at least five such areas in metro Denver, and more are opening in 2001.

I've selected the four best of these areas; all give dogs plenty of room to frolic off leash. Of these four, two are exceptional "dog heavens"—large areas in Chatfield State Park and Cherry Creek Dam State Park. The third superior off-leash area is in Jefferson County Open Space, at the south end of Elk Meadow Open Space Park in Evergreen. The fourth is a three-acre lot in Highlands Ranch, a community where smaller, neighborhood off-leash areas are being planned together with larger, community "dog parks." This spot is next to Redstone Park and takes you through a charming rural area along the High Line Canal.

A final "dog heaven," the wonderful Washington Park, doesn't provide any dog training areas; your companion must remain leashed. I've included it in this section, however, because of its popularity among dog lovers. It's a great place to meet other dog companions and let your pet socialize with his peers. Some local residents are lobbying to change the leash laws here, but at press time giving your dog free rein remains against the law; people are frequently fined for violations.

Dog Heavens

Off-leash areas, aka dog parks, have been around for twenty or so years and are particularly popular in urban and suburban areas where people and their pets are concentrated. However, all off-leash areas have rules, which are usually posted on a sign or listed in a flyer or a brochure put out by the governing municipality. Below is a compendium of these rules:

- You must pick up after your dog.

- You must carry a leash and be inside the off-leash area with your pet.

- Aggressive dogs, dogs in season, and puppies (usually less than four months old) are not permitted.

- Dogs must be vaccinated.

- An adult must supervise children.

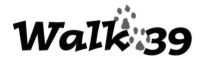

Chatfield State Park

General location: The northeast corner of Chatfield State Park.

Special attractions: Two ponds, a meadow, and picnic areas.

Open: The park is open year-round, but facilities such as the marina and horse stables operate April through October 9 A.M. to 5 P.M.

Total distance: 0.75 to 1.25 miles, depending on the loop you take.

Estimated time: 1 hour.

Services: Rest rooms (closed during the winter months) at the parking lot.

Restrictions: You'll need a daily pass or an annual permit to enter the park. Dogs must be on a leash on the park grounds except in the training area.

For more information: Chatfield State Park, (303) 791–7275.

Getting started

From C–470 south of Denver, take the Wadsworth Boulevard exit. Go south on Wadsworth Boulevard (C–121) to the marked turnoff for Chatfield State Park. Turn left and proceed to the park entrance. After leaving the entrance booth, continue to a stop sign. Turn left and drive for 2 miles, across the dam, to the Stevens Grove parking lot. The dog training area is on your left.

You can also access the park and the dog training area on foot without paying the daily access fee (which is charged for automobile entry). Take the Santa Fe Drive exit off C–470 and head south on Santa Fe for 0.3 mile. At the first traffic light (Blakeland Drive), turn right. Go another 0.3 mile on Blakeland, then turn right onto Riverview Parkway. Take this heavily trafficked industrial road to

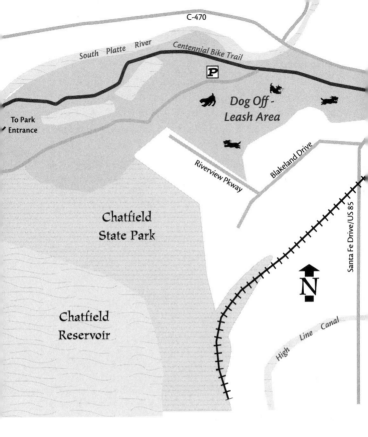

where it dead-ends next to the Amcor Precast Concrete plant. A metal gate provides access to the state park and has the park's symbol on it. There is limited parking on the right for several cars. Go past the gate on a gravel path. The dog training area is about 100 yards ahead of you.

Overview

Chatfield State Park offers a lot—a lake for boating, sailing, and fishing; horse rentals; sandy beaches; marinas; miles of hiking trails; and, yes, an expansive training area, where your dog can swim, wallow, and frolic off the leash to his heart's content.

The walk

🦴 The dog training area consists of two loops around two large ponds. There's also a large meadow that ends in a stand of tall cottonwoods, which provide cool shade on a hot day. The trail around the lake to the left starts out paved, but as it follows the shoreline, it becomes a narrow dirt path. The trail around the pond to the right is paved. On the north side of the lake, the trail intersects with a portion of the C–470 paved trail that's popular among bicyclists.

The meadow southeast of the lake is crisscrossed with dirt paths and is also part of the dog training area. The meadow ends in a second picnic area called Cottonwood Grove.

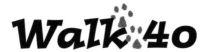

Walk 40

Cherry Creek State Park

General location: Aurora

Special attractions: Fabulous views, and a huge area where your dog can run free.

Open: 6 A. M. to 9 P. M.

Total distance: 1.8 miles round trip.

Estimated time: As long as you and Rover want to frolic.

Services: Rest rooms, water, and a covered picnic area.

Restrictions: Leave no trace after yourself and your dog.

For more information: Cherry Creek State Park, (303) 699–3860.

Getting started

From I–225, take the Parker Road heading south and drive for 1.1 miles to East Lehigh Avenue, which is the entrance to the park. Turn right (west) and continue for 0.6 mile to the entrance booth. Pay a $4 daily fee if you don't have a park pass. (An additional $3 assessment above and beyond the annual park pass is also charged at Cherry Creek. The money is being used to combat algae in the reservoir. You get a decal for the $3 that is good all year.)

Drive for 0.1 mile and take the first left after leaving the booth, then continue for 1.1 miles to another left marked with a sign for the dog training area. After passing the 12-Mile House picnic area, continue for a few hundred more feet to a circular parking area. Park here. The dog training area is 500 yards to the southeast and clearly marked. Your dog must be on a leash until you get there.

Overview

The Cherry Creek State Park dog training area is truly a dog heaven. Stretching for almost a mile, it offers several trails, a huge prairie

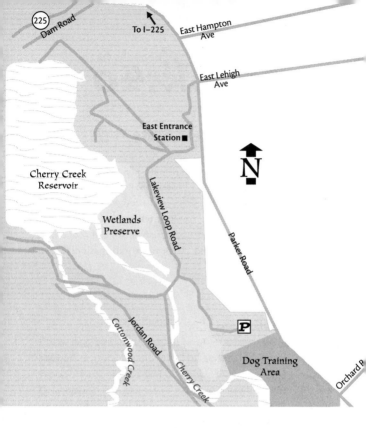

meadow, shady spots under cottonwoods, and numerous access points to the sandy, flat creekbed. Dogs love it here and even if a handful of strangers meet on the path, the animals are invariably well behaved. For the dogs' human companions, there are two benches strategically placed in the shade of cottonwoods from which the Front Range vistas are spectacular.

The walk

🦴 The training area is marked by signs and begins on the south side of a rail fence. A packed-dirt jeep road leads south through

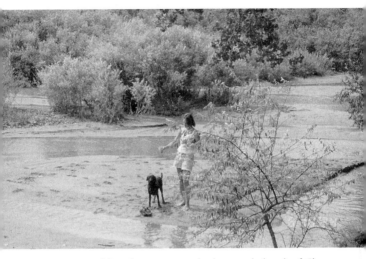

An owner and her dog cavort on the low sandy beach of Cherry Creek.

the middle of the area for 0.3 mile. Wetlands of cattails and willows are to the west; these are off limits to your dog and are clearly marked.

The jeep road trail ends at the bank of Cherry Creek. Take a narrow trail left (east) that follows the creek. There is a bench here under a cottonwood that grows at a strange acute angle. This is one of several easy access points to the creek, which is shallow and spills over a flat, sandy bottom—a great place for a dog to retrieve a thrown ball or a Frisbee while splashing in shallow water.

Continue for another 0.4 mile until the trail crosses the paved path that runs south to north through the park. The park boundary is a few dozen feet on the south side of the paved path. A bench offers great Front Range views. Return the way you came, taking time to stop for another frolic in the water.

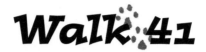

Elk Meadow Park

General location: Evergreen.

Special attractions: A meadow, an aspen stand, and a mountain stream.

Open: One hour before sunrise to one hour after sunset.

Total distance: 1.2 mile round trip.

Estimated time: 30 to 40 minutes.

Services: Rest rooms, water fountains, and picnic tables.

Restrictions: Your dog must be on a leash except in the designated dog training area.

For more information: Jefferson County Open Space, (303) 271–5925.

Getting started

From I–70, take exit 252 (Evergreen) and drive for 6 miles on Evergreen Parkway (C–74) to Stagecoach Boulevard. Turn right (west) and drive for 1.2 miles to the Elk Meadow parking lot, on your right. Park here, or continue another 0.3 mile to a small, two-vehicle pullout on the left (south) side of the road. It's marked by an overgrown jeep road and an opening in the wire fence.

Overview

The dog training area stretches from the south side of Stagecoach Road to the park's boundaries. It's a tall grass meadow bisected by a trail, a stand of aspen on the south side, and a small mountain stream that descends rather steeply into a gulch to the park boundary (clearly marked by fences and signs).

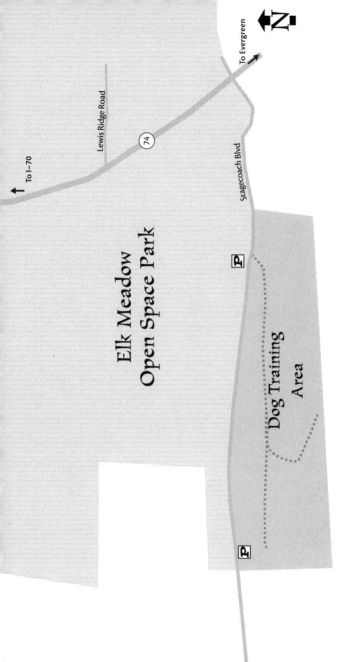

The walk

🦴If you parked at the large, paved parking lot, cross Stagecoach Road carefully. Signs and a narrow trail lead to the dog training area 0.25 mile to the west. The trail follows the road until it reaches the meadow and a trail that branches off to the left.

🦴If you parked at the small turnoff, enter through the opening in the fence and turn left (east) to access the larger trail through the field.

🦴Follow the trail across the meadow and into the trees. There is no bridge over the small, narrow creek; you cross the creek by stepping over the channel. Follow the trail down and to the left as it follows the gulch. The banks of the creek grow steeper the farther down you go. The trail ends in 0.3 mile at a wire fence designated private land.

🦴Turn around and return the way you came.

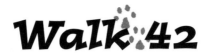

Walk 42

Highlands Ranch

General location: Highlands Ranch in Douglas County.

Special attractions: A community dog off-leash area near the High Line Canal.

Open: Sunrise to sunset.

Total distance: The area covers three acres.

Estimated time: As long as you and your dog wish to romp.

Services: Rest rooms, water and a playground across the street in Redstone Park; picnic tables inside the fenced-off area.

Restrictions: Pick up after your pet.

For more information: Highlands Ranch Metropolitan Districts, (303) 791–2710

Getting started

From C–470, take the Lucent Boulevard exit and go south on Lucent Boulevard for 0.6 mile to its intersection with Town Center Drive. Make a right (west) onto Town Center Drive, and continue for 0.8 mile to its intersection with Foothills Canyon Boulevard. Turn left and park in the parking lot on your right, just past the tennis courts.

Overview

Highland Ranch is one of the newest suburbs in the Denver metro area, and its development of parks and other outdoor amenities is still ongoing. A community survey conducted in 1999 showed that residents rank the addition of dog off-leash areas third in importance among outdoor amenities; only adding more hard- and soft-surface trails ranked higher than the desire for dog parks. Construction of "Hound Hill" next to Redstone Park addressed this

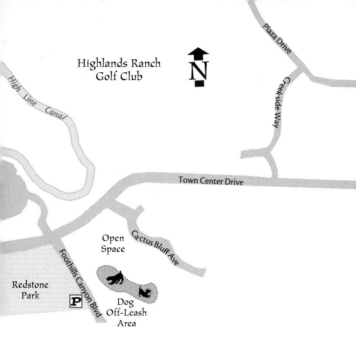

resident request. This off-leash area opened in 2000. It's the first of two large community dog parks, that will be augmented by smaller, neighborhood off-leash areas.

The training area

Park your vehicle and leash your dog. Cross the street and head for the gate to the fenced dog training area. Once you're inside the three-acre dirt lot, take off the leash and let your dog head for the whimsical fire hydrant in the middle of the park.

There's a picnic table at which you can sit while Rover enjoys his freedom. Trees planted around the perimeter of the lot will eventually provide shade. If you'd like a little more exercise, consider taking your pet on a walk along the High Line Canal, which is across Town Center Drive (see Walk 2).

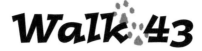

Walk 43

Washington Park

General location: Central Denver.

Special attractions: A park with numerous facilities, two lakes, a recreation center, and beautiful flower plantings during the growing season. It's a great place for dog- and people-watching.

Open: 6 A.M. to 11 P.M.

Total distance: 0.6 mile around Smith Lake; just under 1 mile around Grasmere Lake; 2.6 miles on the crushed-gravel trail around the perimeter of the park; and 2.2 miles on the inner road, which is closed to traffic except where it provides access to in-park parking lots.

Estimated time: 25 minutes around Smith Lake; 40 minutes around Grasmere Lake.

Services: Portable toilets are scattered around the park, as are playgrounds, picnic tables, and playing fields. Fishing in the two lakes is permitted with a valid Colorado fishing license. Telephones and water fountains can be found near park buildings.

Restrictions: Your dog must be on a leash. Curb your pet, pick up after him, and dispose of waste. Disposal plastic bags are provided at many locations throughout the park.

For more information: Denver Parks and Recreation Department, (303) 698–4903

Getting started

Washington Park is centrally located, south of downtown and southwest of the Cherry Creek shopping area, so it can be reached from several major streets. If you're unfamiliar with its location, the easiest access is to take exit 206A (Downing Street) off I-25 and go north on Downing for 2 blocks. On the south, the park begins

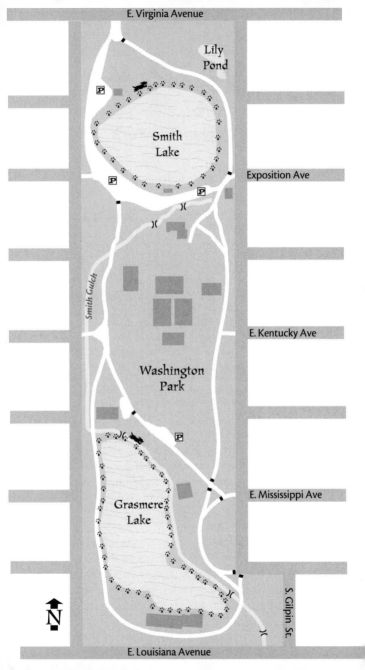

at East Louisiana Avenue, stretching north 8 blocks to East Virginia Avenue. It's 4 blocks wide.

You can also reach Washington Park by going east from South Broadway on East Exposition Avenue. Or head west from South University Boulevard, also on Exposition (or on another parallel street). There's parking on nearby streets, and limited parking in the park itself on the west and south sides of Smith Lake and the northeast side of Grasmere Lake.

Overview

Washington Park is to Denverites what Central Park is to Manhattanites. It's a lovely park with mature trees and wide grassy expanses and two lakes that are annually stocked for fishing. The 160-acre park was designed in 1899.

Washington Park is heavily used for all manner of recreation, ranging from indoor use of the Washington Park Recreation Center to walking, jogging, in-line skating, fishing, ball playing, sunning, picnicking, dog walking and people-watching.

The park is traversed by Smith Ditch (aka City Ditch), one of the earliest irrigation projects in the area. In 1860 the government of the Kansas Territory authorized the Capital Hydraulic Company to build the irrigation project. The project ran into financial problems and was completed by John W. Smith, for whom it and the nearby lake are named. In the 1870s the ditch was acquired by the city; it provides irrigation water to Washington Park's two lakes, along with the Denver Country Club and City Park. Smith Ditch was added to the National Register of Historic Places in 1977. A plaque commemorating the event is located just west of the recreation center on the banks of the ditch.

Before the arrival of settlers, Washinton Park's Smith Lake was a buffalo wallow on the prairie. With the establishment of Denver, it became the city's first bathing beach. The Dos Chappell Bathhouse is the structure on the northwest side of Smith Lake. The bathhouse was built in 1912 for $10,000 to serve as a changing room for bathers in summer and a warming house for skaters in winter. Smith Lake was closed to bathing in 1957 due to a polio scare. Subsequently, the building fell into disrepair. In the early 1990s Dos Chappell, a Colorado native and local resident, led the effort to restore the building; it was named in his honor in 1996.

There are several other structures in the park, including the boathouse pavilion, also restored, on the south side of Smith Lake, and the Washington Park Recreation Center, off South Franklin Street at East Exposition Avenue.

The Eugene Field House, a small building at the East Exposition Entrance to the park, is also on the National Register of Historic Places. The home of Eugene Field when he lived in Denver in the 1880s, it was moved to the park in 1930 from its original location at 397 Colfax Avenue.

Grasmere Lake is the larger of the park's two lakes. It's a favorite locale for walking dogs. Although dogs are not permitted in either lake, many people do let their pets go in. Know that the area is patrolled, and if your dog shows signs of having been in the water, you'll be fined. Fines are also assessed for letting your dog off leash.

Flower and garden aficionados should not miss the annual plantings along Downing Street between Ohio and Exposition Avenues. A covered display board behind the plantings identifies the flowers and their location in the numerous beds. Another large planting of annuals is located near the East Mississippi Avenue entrance on the east side of the park. This garden follows the pattern of plantings at Mount Vernon, George Washington's home. Adjacent are the bowling green and club offices of the Washington Lawn Bowling Club, established in 1925. In warm weather local rugby and soccer clubs often hold tournaments in the numerous ball fields on the east side of the park, between Tennessee and Ohio Avenues.

A paved road winds around the park, but many of its segments are closed to vehicular traffic. The road is mostly used by bikers and in-line skaters, so it's not the best place to walk your dog. An exception is the segment on the west side of Grasmere Lake; one lane here is dedicated to pedestrians. The narrow asphalt paths around both lakes are suitable for a walk with your dog.

The park is the home of sizable flock of Canada geese, and it's a migration stop for other waterfowl. Many signs warn park users against feeding or harassing wildlife.

The walks

🦴 **Smith Lake Loop:** After parking on the street or at the northwest or south parking lots at Smith Lake, put your dog on a leash and walk down to the paved trail that goes around the lake. It's 0.6 mile long. If you started at the northwest parking lot near the Dos Chappell Bathhouse, go past the building and continue along the shoreline. As you reach the east side of the lake, you'll see Lily Pond on your left. It's restricted to fishing by young people fifteen years and younger. No fishing license is required. Lily Pond and Smith and Grasmere Lakes are under the jurisdiction of the Colorado Division of Wildlife. As you walk on the east side of the lake, notice the view of the Front Range to the west, beyond the tall elms and cottonwoods. Complete your walk by going past the boathouse pavilion and playground on the south side of the lake.

🦴 **Grasmere Lake Loop:** After parking on the street or along East Mississippi Avenue, off South Franklin Street, inside the park, put your dog on a leash and walk down to the paved trail that goes around the lake. It's 0.96 mile long. If you began at the Mississippi parking area, note the large beds of seasonal flowers that you'll pass on your way to the lake. Near the plantings are two small pedestrian bridges across Smith Ditch, which flows along the north and east sides of Grasmere Lake before crossing East Louisiana Avenue. Once you reach the lake, continue south, then west past the tennis courts and in the shade of tall deciduous trees and conifers. The path narrows on the west side of the lake, so you might like to access the paved road that parallels it. The road is closed to vehicles, and the lane nearest you is dedicated to pedestrian traffic. As you reach the north shore of the lake, you'll pass several horseshoe pits and a basketball court. Complete your walk at one of the footbridges over Smith Ditch.

Appendix A

Park Agencies and Organizations

Adams County Department of
Parks and Community Resources
977 Henderson Road
Brighton, CO 80610
(303) 637–8000

Adams County Trail Rangers
7265 Birch Street
Commerce City, CO 80022
(303) 637–8000

Aurora Parks and Open Space
Department
1470 South Havana
Aurora, CO 80012
(303) 739–7160

Barr Lake State Park
13401 Picadilly Road
Brighton, CO 80601
(303) 659–6005
e-mail: barrlake@csn.net

Bear Creek Lake Park
15600 West Morrison Road
Morrison, CO 80465
(303) 697–6159

Boulder County Parks and
Open Space
2045 Thirteenth Street
Boulder, CO 80202
(303) 441–3950

Chatfield State Park
11500 North Roxborough Park
Road
Littleton, CO 80125
Office: (303) 791–7275
Marina: (303) 791–5555
Livery: (303) 933–3636
e-mail: chatfld@csn.net

Cherry Creek State Park
4201 South Parker Road
Aurora, CO 80014
(303) 699–3860
e-mail: chycrk@csn.net

Colorado State Parks
1313 Sherman Street, Room 618
Denver, CO 80203
(303) 866–3437
www.parks.state.co.us

Denver Water Department
1600 West Twelfth Avenue
Denver, CO 80204
(303) 628–6170
Community Relations Office:
(303) 628–6324
Recreation Office:
(303) 628–6526
Denver Water has published *The
Guide to the High Line Canal*, a

pocket-sized booklet, available at Denver bookstores and through the agency for $4.50.

Denver Parks and Recreation Department (Trails)
2300 Fifteenth Street
Denver, CO 80202
(303) 698–4903

Four Mile House Historic Park
715 South Forest Street
Denver, CO 80222
(303) 399–1859

Golden Gate Canyon State Park
3873 Highway 46
Golden, CO 80403
(303) 582–3707
e-mail: goldgate@csn.net

Highlands Ranch Metropolitan Districts
62 West Plaza Drive
Highlands Ranch, CO 89126
(303) 791–2710

Jefferson County Open Space
700 Jefferson County Parkway
Suite 100
Golden, CO 80401
(303) 271–5925

South Suburban Park and Recreation District
6631 South University Boulevard
Littleton, CO 80121
(303) 789–5131

South Platte River Greenway Foundation
1666 South University Boulevard
Suite B
Denver, CO 80210
(303) 698–1322

City of Thornton Parks Department
2211 Eppinger Boulevard
Thornton, CO 80229
(303) 538–7632

Appendix B

Dog-Friendly Organizations

Colorado Greyhound Adoption, Inc., P.O. Box 2404, Littleton, CO 80161–2404; (303) 816–2799 or 1–800–366–1472; www.greyhound adoption.com. The CGA is a non-profit organization devoted to placement and adoption of greyhounds.

Colorado Humane Society & S.P.C.A., Inc. This is the oldest ongoing corporation in Colorado and one of the oldest humane societies in the United States. Founded in 1881, it assists animal care organizations throughout Colorado. The society has two locations. The "no-kill" shelter is located at 2760 South Platte River Drive, Englewood, CO 80110; (303) 781–9344. The veterinary hospital is at 1864 South Wadsworth Blvd. #7, Lakewood, CO 80232; (303) 988–4465. The website address is www.coloradohumane.org where you can also find web links to other Colorado organizations that help or protect animals.

Dalmatian Rescue of Colorado, Inc., 6828 Rim Rock Trail, Fort Collins, CO 80526. This is a non-profit organization dedicated to locating permanent homes for unwanted or abandoned Dalmatians. The group coordinates rescue activities throughout Colorado, Wyoming, Idaho, and New Mexico, and provides consultation services to assist Dalmatian owners. Dalmatian Rescue sponsors events throughout the year to raise funds. The group sponsors an annual Agility Day in the spring in which dogs of all breeds and their owners can compete. To get more information on an upcoming event, call the Dalmatian Rescue Hotline (303) 415–5703 or visit www.dalmatianrescue.org.

Dumb Friends League, 2080 South Quebec Street, Denver, CO 80231-3298; (303) 696–4941. Founded in 1910, the Denver Dumb Friends League places homeless pets with new families, investigates reports of animal cruelty and reunites lost pets with their owners. The league also gives free education presentations; provides animal behavior assistance to prospective, new, and experienced pet owners; and offers free referrals for pet-friendly rental housing. It also sponsors the PEDIGREE Furry Scurry the first weekend in May in Washington Park. Additional information, as well as links to other animal organizations, is available at www.ddfl.org.

Humane Society of Boulder Valley, 2323 Fifty-fifth Street, Boulder, CO; (303) 442–4030 and (303) 442–4030. This is arguably the most proactive animal shelter along the Front Range. It interviews prospective adoptive families and has been known to turn some down. The society sponsors a popular fundraiser in September that involves a walk with your pet. The society can be reached also by e-mail at humane@boulderhumane.org and www.boulderhumane.org.

Lifeline Puppy Rescue is a no kill shelter for young puppies. The hotline is (303) 655-9696. The group's website features photos of puppies available for adoption and success stories about placed dogs. The Internet address is www.lifelinepuppy.org.

The Longmont Humane Society, 9595 Nelson Road, Longmont, CO 80501; (303) 772–1232. LHS is a private, non-profit organization dedicated to the protection of animals. It provides temporary shelter to lost, abandoned or surrendered domesticated and wild animals. It sponsors several dog-related events each year, including a dog walk in the spring. More information is available at info@longmonthumane.org. The web address is www.longmont humane.org.

MaxFund Animal Adoption Center, 1025 Galapago Street, Denver, CO 80204, (303) 595–4917. The Max Fund is a no-kill shelter for injured animals with no known owners. The shelter cares for stray, cast-off, and orphan cats and dogs found on the streets of Denver city and county, and finds homes for these animals. The fund is named after a stray dog that was injured on I–25 but was rescued. Donations for Max's care resulted in the creation of the fund in 1987. MaxFund also sponsors low-cost spay and neuter clinics and vaccination clinics, and donates food to the homeless for their own pets.

Star Fire Dog Adoption Inc., P.O. Box 16207, Golden, CO 80402-6004; (303) 642–9233. This organization places dogs of owners who are entering a nursing home or are terminally ill. The organization can also be reached at info@starfiredogadoption.com and at www.starfiredogadoption.com.

Appendix C

Annual Dog Events

Washington Park hosts the **PEDIGREE Furry Scurry** the first weekend in May. This is *the* social event for dogs in the Denver metro area. The event is a pledge walk/run that raises money for the Denver Dumb Friends League. The course is around one of the lakes and is about 2 miles. If you like, bring your dog, or walk or run in honor of your favorite pet. For further information, contact the league at (303) 696–4941 or www.ddfl.org/events. There is an entry fee, which is reduced when registering by mid-April. If you bring your dog, your pet must wear current identification and rabies vaccination tags and be on a 6-foot or shorter leash at all times.

Agility Day Fundraiser is an annual indoor obstacle course for dogs and their owners that is sponsored by Dalmatian Rescue of Colorado. If your dog excels in tricks and acrobatics this event is a great opportunity for you and your pet to make new friends and try out the obstacle course, which consists of barrels, low jumps, and the like. The event is held in the spring and indoors at Pets Control, 876 Ventura Street in Aurora, off the Sixth Avenue exit off I-225. The participation fee is a $5.00 donation per dog (tax deductible). Participating dogs must be on a leash and the pet should be current on shots. Call the Dalmatian Rescue Hotline (303) 415–5703 to make sure that the event will take place or visit www.dalmatianrescue.org.

The Longmont Humane Society sponsors an annual **3-mile pledge walk** in late spring to raise funds for its shelter. The event features booths and other activities. Get more information by calling the society at (303) 772–1232 or visiting www.longmonthumane.org

A **Frisbee canine tournament** in which you and your pet can compete is a regular feature of the annual Western Welcome

Week, held at Arapahoe Community College, off Santa Fe Drive in Littleton, the second two weeks in August. The canine Frisbee event is sponsored by The QUADRUPED and is a disc catching competition. Additional information is available by calling Western Welcome Week at (303) 759–8785 and by visiting www.TheQuadruped.com.

The Boulder Humane Society sponsors an annual **4-mile walk along Boulder Creek** in early September. The walk begins and ends in downtown Boulder and is the local social event for dogs and their owners. Participants collect pledges that are contributed to the society. Booths and entertainment are also featured during the daylong event. Additional information can be obtained by calling the society at (303) 442–4030.

Acknowledgments

Dog lovers know the places dogs love most, and many have shared with me their favorite locales during casual encounters on many trails in the metro Denver area. Special thanks are due the several rangers in the Jefferson County Open Space program, who were knowledgeable about the terrain in the foothills and about dog-friendly trails. I'm also indebted to the members of the Colorado Mountain Club, who participate in "doggie hikes" for companionship and "tall dog tales."

Thomas J. Hoby, director of parks and open space for the Highlands Ranch Metro Districts, shared information on a survey his agency did that showed that dog off-leash areas were one of the three expanded park amenities that local residents most want. Ruth Murayama, a landscape architect with the Denver Department of Parks and Recreation, provided maps and plans for two of Denver's newest riverside parks, and Chad Anderson, Denver Parks and Recreation Department, provided insights on trails along the greenbelts. Robert Carroll and Randy Jacobs, both with the Aurora Planning Department, and Michael F. Turner, prinicpal planner with the Aurora Parks and Open Space Department, helped with mapping the walks in that city. Crystal Gray, director of parks in Adams County, supplied updates on the construction of the Platte River Greenway in Adams County; Michelle Radice, recreation specialist with the Denver Water Department, offered historical background on the High Line Canal.

Jean Flynn and Melissa Reese-Thacker from the South Suburban Park and Recreation District offered assistance with mapping the High Line Canal walks. Kent Wiley, manager of Chatfield State Park, and Robert C. Bruce, project manager, Colorado State Parks, helped with trails in state-operated metro-area parks. Amy Pulver, executive director of the Sand Creek Regional Greenway, offered updates on the development of that greenbelt. Jeff Shoemaker, executive director of the Platte River Greenway, offered pointers about

Denver's oldest greenbelt. Sue Shafer provided information about trails around Bluff Lake, and Megan Davis from Boulder County Parks and Open Space supplied updates on the changes at Rock Creek Farm.

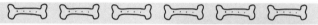

About the Author

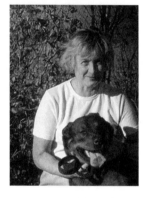

M. A. Savage moved to Denver in the early 1980s and settled near the High Line Canal, which she has been walking ever since. She is an active member of the Colorado Mountain Club. In preparing this book, she hiked more than 300 miles on Denver's greenbelts and in the foothills.

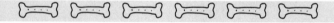